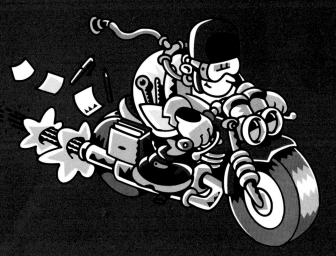

Psychiatry

Series editor
Wilfred Yeo
BMedSci, MB, ChB, MD, MRCP
Senior Lecturer in Medicine,
Medicine/Clinical
Pharmacology and
Therapeutics,
University of
Sheffield

Faculty advisor
MJ Akhtar
MSc, MBBS, DPM,
FRCPsych
Honorary Lecturer,
Newcastle University
Consultant Psychiatrist,
South Tyneside Health
Care Trust,
South Shields

Psychiatry

Darran Bloye
BM, MRCPsych
Sheffield and North Trent
Psychiatry Rotation
Sheffield

Simon Davies
MA (Oxon), MBBS
Research Registrar
Clinical Pharmacology and
Therapeutics
University of Sheffield

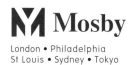

M Mosby

London • Philadelphia
St Louis • Sydney • Tokyo

Editor	**Louise Crowe**
Development Editor	**Filipa Maia**
Project Manager	**Louise Patchett**
Designer	**Greg Smith**
Layout	**Rob Curran**
Illustration Management	**Danny Pyne**
Illustrators	**Debra Woodward**
	Jeremy Theobald
Cover Design	**Greg Smith**
Production	**Susan Walby**
Index	**Janine Ross**

ISBN 0 7234 3140 X

Published by Mosby, an imprint of Mosby International Ltd, Lynton House, 7–12 Tavistock Square, London WC1H 9LB, UK.

Printed by GraphyCems, Navarra, Spain, 1998.
Text set in Crash Course–VAG Light; captions in Crash Course–VAG Thin.

Cataloguing in Publication Data
A catalogue record for this book is available from the British Library.

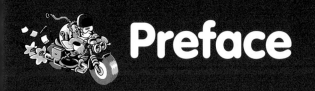

Preface

At first glance psychiatry may seem complex, perhaps even mysterious, and certainly rather different from other medical specialities. In *Crash Course Psychiatry*, we aim to make the subject more approachable, using case vignettes, bulleted lists for easy reference, and hints and tips boxes which highlight key facts. We illustrate how, as in other specialities, patients may present with a wide variety of symptoms and how taking a full history and performing an examination (in particular a mental state examination) lead ultimately to a diagnosis and to treatment.

In Part I, sixteen of the most common presentations in psychiatry are considered. Each chapter begins with a case vignette, enabling readers to focus on patients' presenting complaints whatever the actual diagnosis. Following the cases are definitions of all symptoms and signs (psychopathology) related to the main complaint. We consider differential diagnoses and how to distinguish between them, finally returning to the vignette to discuss the most likely diagnosis.

Part II provides concise information on assessing psychiatric patients and on treatments with drugs and psychotherapy. We return to specific psychiatric disorders and the main sub-specialities in Part III, with essential background information on aetiology, epidemiology, investigations and management. Finally, there is a self assessment section with multiple-choice and short-answer questions, and patient management problems which may be used for group discussion.

One obvious difference between psychiatry and many other branches of medicine is that diagnoses rarely rely on simple laboratory or radiological tests. For this reason, international committees have produced guidelines for diagnosing psychiatric conditions according to symptoms and signs. The most commonly used diagnostic systems are the American *Diagnostic and Statistical Manual of Mental Disorders, 4th edition* (DSM-IV) and the World Health Organisation's *International Standard Classification of Diseases and Health Related Problems, 10th revision* (ICD-10). Both of these systems are explained in this book and we have attempted to highlight differences between the two.

This book is primarily aimed at medical students. It may also be helpful for doctors starting off in psychiatry or undertaking a short attachment as part of training for general practice, nurses, occupational therapists, pharmacists, social workers and indeed any involved in the treatment of psychiatric patients.

Simon Davies
Darran Bloye
Sheffield 1998

Preface

Psychiatry is often perceived by medical students as being interesting, but far too complex. While there are many textbooks which assist students in psychiatry, there is no comprehensive and compact volume of psychiatry. *Crash Course Psychiatry* is a welcome effort to meet this need. It presents essential basic knowledge of psychiatry in a simple, clear and concise manner with the aid of tables and bulleted lists which promote understanding and retention of information.

The text has been carefully selected to reflect the educational needs of students and is presented in a readable format. *Crash Course Psychiatry* takes a problem orientated approach which is based on good clinical practice. At the end of the book is a self-assessment section that focuses on commonly asked examination topics enabling students to test their knowledge and assess their performance through multiple-choice and short-answer questions, and patient management problems.

Crash Course Psychiatry will be invaluable to both medical students and junior doctors. It is hoped that it will be widely used as an aid for effective revision and to supplement standard textbooks.

M. J. Akhtar
Faculty Advisor

So you have an exam in medicine and you don't know where to start? The answer is easy—start with *Crash Course*. Medicine is fun to learn if you can bring it to life with patients who need their problems solving. Conventional medical textbooks are written back-to-front, starting with the diagnosis and then describing the disease. This is because medicine evolved by careful observations and descriptions of individual diseases for which, until this century, there was no treatment. Modern medicine is about problem solving, learning methods to find the right path through the differential diagnosis, and offering treatment promptly.

This series of books has been designed to help you solve common medical problems by starting with the patient and extracting the salient points in the history, examination and investigations. Part II gives you essential information on the physical examination and investigations as seen through the eyes of practising doctors in their specialty. Once the diagnosis is made, you can refer to Part III to confirm that the diagnosis is correct and get advice regarding treatment.

Throughout the series we have included informative diagrams and hints and tips boxes to simplify your learning. The books are meant as revision tools, but are comprehensive, accurate and well balanced and should enable you to learn each subject well. To check that you did learn something from the book, (rather than just flashing it in front of your eyes!), we have added a self-assessment section in the usual format of most medical exams—multiple-choice and short-answer questions (with answers), and patient management problems for self-directed learning. Good luck!

Wilf Yeo
Series Editor (Clinical)

Contents

Contents

Acknowledgements

We would like to acknowledge the help and support from our colleagues in Sheffield, especially Dr Brendan Murphy for his advice on the manuscript and to Dr Chris Lawson, Dr Chris Wallbridge, Dr Miguel Fernandez, Dr Martin Lennard, Dr Andrew Bowen and Mr Peter Pratt. We also wish to thank Ms Giovanna Battiston and Dr Rachel Clarke.

This book is dedicated to Gianna and Maureen Cheshire (x2)

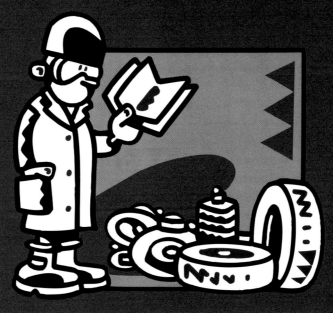

THE PATIENT PRESENTS WITH

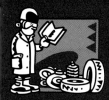

1. Low and Elevated Mood

Mrs LM, a 32-year-old married housewife with two children aged 4 and 6 years, presented to her family doctor stating that she was persistently unhappy and had been crying repeatedly over the past few weeks. She had no previous psychiatric history and had moved to the area 3 years earlier when her husband was promoted. She appeared to have integrated well into the neighbourhood at first, involving herself in the organization of a toddlers' group. Unfortunately, the group had dissolved a few months ago when her co-organizer and only close confidante had moved away. Deprived of her most important social outlet, Mrs LM had found herself more dominated by her young children and felt she lacked the motivation to keep in touch with the other mothers from the group. She had begun to feel persistently tired, often wakening early in the morning, and had gained over a stone in weight, having turned to food for comfort. She told her family doctor that in the last month she had felt particularly worthless because she was too tired to look after the children. She felt guilty for letting her husband down, as she was too miserable to feel attractive and had lost interest in the sexual aspects of their relationship. There appeared to be no relief from her unhappiness—no aspect of her life gave her pleasure and she found herself crying spontaneously whenever she was on her own.

Psychopathology
Mood and affect

The term 'mood' describes a sustained state of emotion in relation to the surroundings. Both low and elevated mood reflect pathological changes in this relationship, and the changes may be subjective or objective (i.e. reported by the patient or by others). In depression, the mood may be profoundly sad and despondent, but sometimes is marked only by disinterest and apathy. The term 'affect' (as in 'affective disorders') refers to a more transient observed expression of emotion. Thus, low mood is often associated with affective flattening—an objective reduction in the observed emotional response.

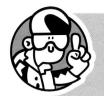

Remember the distinction between the terms 'mood' and 'affect': they are not the same.

Key depressive symptoms that usually accompany low mood are:

- The inability to derive any pleasure from activities that were formerly enjoyed (anhedonia) and loss of interest in such previously pleasurable activities.
- Lack of energy or increased fatiguability.

3

Other symptoms associated with low mood may be considered under the headings cognitive, biological, psychotic, and catatonic symptoms.

Cognitive symptoms
The cognitive symptoms of depression include those listed below.

Poor concentration The tendency to worry repeatedly over existing problems may occur to the extent that the problems intrude into the thoughts at the expense of everything else and make concentrating difficult.

Poor self-esteem The patient with low mood may gain the impression that they have fallen short in their own or others' expectations, or have become a worthless person. They may feel 'useless'.

Guilt Patients with low mood may blame themselves either for an action or omission that has led to undesirable consequences, or for the very act of developing low mood itself and its associated symptoms. The guilt is often inappropriate or out of proportion.

Hopelessness If low mood is severe, sufferers may believe that there is no way out of their current situation.

Biological (or somatic) symptoms
The biological (or somatic) symptoms of depression include those listed below.

Anhedonia (See above.)

Appetite and weight loss Many patients with low mood experience a reduction in appetite and may lose weight. However, some individuals turn to 'comfort eating' and their low mood heralds an increased appetite and corresponding weight gain – these symptoms, however, are not considered biological.

Early morning wakening Although the patient may be able to get to sleep at a reasonable hour, they wake at least two hours earlier than normal (e.g. at 4.30 a.m. rather than 8.30 a.m.) and find it impossible to get back to sleep. Whilst early morning wakening is the most common pattern of sleep disruption, conversely hypersomnia (excess sleep) may occur – but again, this is not considered a biological symptom.

Loss of libido Patients with low mood may report a loss of interest in sexual activities. As in the above vignette, reduction of libido may add further fuel to cognitive symptoms such as guilt when the sufferer feels unable to satisfy their partner.

Diurnal variation of mood Low mood may occur, or be most pronounced, at a specific time of day, often in the morning.

Psychomotor retardation and agitation Movements may be slowed, with the facial movements and gestures that accompany speech diminished and the voice quiet and monotonous. Furthermore, a patient may develop agitation and an inability to sit still, with hand wringing, tapping, and other signs of frustration or impatience.

Reduced emotional reactivity Events which would normally produce a response are reacted to with less emotion.

Be sure to know the biological symptoms of depression very well: they are often asked for in exams!

Psychotic symptoms
In severe depressive episodes, patients may experience disorders of thought-content, including delusions, and of perception, including hallucinations, which are explained fully in Chapter 5. Delusions and hallucinations associated with depression are most often 'mood congruent', i.e. their content is in line with the low mood. For instance, delusions may consist of feelings that the world is black, the mind frozen, or the body wasting away. There may also be a delusional sense of guilt, worthlessness, or wickedness. Hallucinations may take the form of voices criticizing the subject in the second person.

Catatonic symptoms
Catatonic features occur rarely, appearing only in the severely depressed patient. They are described in Chapter 13.

Suicidal ideation

Low mood, especially when accompanied by poor self-esteem, guilt, and hopelessness, may lead to thoughts of ending one's life. Such thoughts may be fleeting and rejected quickly or they may persist and lead to the formation of a suicide plan. Suicidal activity is discussed fully in Chapter 12.

Differential diagnosis

Depression

In ICD-10, depression is referred to more formally as 'depressive episode'; in DSM-IV it appears as 'major depressive episode'.

To meet the ICD-10 criteria, it is necessary to have at least 2 weeks of suffering at least two of the core symptoms of depression, these being:

- Lowering of mood to an extent that is abnormal for the individual.
- Reduction in energy.
- A loss of interest in, or enjoyment of, normally pleasurable activities.

To clinch the diagnosis of a depressive episode, some of the following symptoms need also to be present:

- Loss of confidence.
- Feelings of guilt.
- Thoughts of suicide.
- Poor concentration.
- Changed sleep.
- Changed appetite.
- Agitation or retardation.

A mild depressive episode has a total of four symptoms from these two lists; a moderate episode, at least six; and the threshold for a severe depressive episode is eight, including all three core symptoms.

Severe episodes may be described as having psychotic features when delusions or hallucinations are present.

To fulfil the DSM-IV criteria for a major depressive episode requires five symptoms from a similar list, one of which must be 'depressed mood' or 'loss of interest or pleasure'. A 2-week duration is again needed and symptoms must cause a clinically significant loss of social or occupational functioning.

Recurrent depressive disorder

As mood disorders often occur repeatedly, the diagnosis of recurrent depressive disorder has been established for patients with two or more episodes of depression.

Dysthymia

Dysthymia involves chronic and prolonged depressed mood which may go on for a number of years but is hardly ever sufficiently severe to satisfy formally the criteria for a depressive episode. ICD-10 requires only three symptoms from a list that includes tearfulness, pessimism, despair, and social withdrawal, as well as many of the symptoms that appear under 'depressive episode'.

Bipolar affective disorder

Depressive disorders are unipolar: mood is either low or normal. When periods of both elevated and low mood have occurred, the disorder is considered bipolar, as mood has diverged from normal towards both poles. Bipolar disorders are discussed in the second part of this chapter.

Adjustment disorder

Low mood may appear as one of several symptoms that arises when a subject has had to adapt to a significant change in life. When it can be confidently assumed that the symptoms would not have arisen without the stress due to the life event, the diagnosis of adjustment disorder is applied (see Chapter 4). Bereavement, where low mood and other symptoms typical of depression and anxiety are provoked by the death of a significant person, is a form of adjustment reaction.

Depression secondary to psychiatric or general medical disorders or to psychoactive substances

Low mood and associated depressive symptoms may be primary (occurring in the absence of or predating other disorders), or secondary to other psychiatric or organic problems. For example, an individual who has schizophrenia, dementia, an anxiety disorder, or an eating disorder may go on to experience secondary depression as a consequence. General medical conditions which may produce secondary depression through presumed direct chemical effects are listed in Fig. 1.1. Furthermore, any general medical condition that is unpleasant or debilitating may produce secondary depression for psychological reasons.

Depression may occur secondarily to the use of both prescribed (Fig. 1.2) and illicit drugs and to other substances such as alcohol. For example, reserpine, an antihypertensive agent, is thought to produce depression by depletion of presynaptic catecholamine stores. DSM-

General medical conditions causing low mood			
Neurological	**Endocrine**	**Infections**	**Others**
multiple sclerosis Parkinson's disease Huntington's disease spinal cord injury stroke (CVA, especially left anterior infarcts) head injury cerebral tumours	Cushing's disease Addison's disease thyroid disorders (especially hypothyroidism) parathyroid disorders	infectious mononucleiosis herpes simplex brucellosis typhoid HIV/AIDS syphilis	malignancies (especially pancreatic cancer) systemic lupus erythematosus rheumatoid arthritis renal failure porphyria vitamin deficiencies (e.g. niacin)

Fig. 1.1 General medical conditions causing low mood.

Prescribed drugs causing low mood	
Drug group	**Examples**
antihypertensives	reserpine, methyl dopa
steroids	corticosteroids, oral contraceptives
antiparkinsonian	L-dopa
analgesics	opiates

Fig. 1.2 Prescribed drugs causing low mood.

IV includes the diagnosis 'substance-induced mood disorder' for mood change that is specific to the use of, exposure to, or withdrawal from a substance.

Discussion of vignette

What is the most likely diagnosis for Mrs LM?

It is likely that Mrs LM is experiencing a depressive episode. She has low mood sustained for considerably longer than the 2 weeks required, a loss of interest or pleasure in activities that were previously pleasurable, and decreased energy or increased fatiguability. She also has sufficient of the additional symptoms—specifically, loss of confidence, guilt, sleep disturbance, and appetite change—to clinch the diagnosis. This would be considered a moderate depressive episode as seven depressive symptoms are present, including three core symptoms. Note that both cognitive and biological symptoms are represented. There do not appear to be any psychotic symptoms, but Mrs LM must be asked whether features such as hallucinations and delusions have occurred (see Chapter 5).

As this is a first episode, the diagnosis of recurrent depressive disorder is not appropriate. Similarly,

dysthymia is not a suitable diagnosis as the period of low mood is much too short, the severity of the present episode too great, and the deterioration in functioning too marked.

How do we further characterize the history of the episode?

Factors causing and maintaining Mrs LM's low mood should be examined. It is usual to consider the three categories listed in Fig. 1.3.

As an inherited vulnerability to depression may be a key predisposing factor, a family history of mental illness in first-degree relatives should be elicited. Precipitating factors are those events occurring immediately before the onset of low mood; perpetuating factors are those that may be considered to prolong the episode. Often the removal of a perpetuating factor such as unemployment or illness can alleviate a depressive episode.

Does she have primary or secondary depression?

There is no suggestion in Mrs LM's story that her

> **Never forget to ask a patient who complains of low mood whether they have thought of suicide, and if so, whether they have gone as far as formulating a suicide plan.**

depression has developed secondarily to another psychiatric or organic cause. However, a full history and clinical examination should be undertaken to exclude alcohol and substance misuse, general medical conditions (see Fig. 1.1), and other psychiatric disorders (e.g. schizophrenia, obsessive–compulsive disorder, panic disorder).

How do we rule out bipolar affective disorder?

To rule out bipolar affective disorder we need to enquire whether Mrs LM has experienced any significant period of elevated or expansive mood with hypomanic or manic symptoms such as increased talkativeness, overspending, or a decreased need for sleep.

What about an adjustment reaction?

Mrs LM's original move to the district—a notable 'life event'—occurred 3 years ago and did not in itself provoke low mood. The more than 2-year gap before the onset of low mood mitigates against a diagnosis of adjustment disorder.

Predisposing, precipitating and perpetuating factors in Mrs LM's depression	
Factors	**Examples from Mrs LM's history**
predisposing	lack of employment outside the home
precipitating	loss of only close confidante loss of main social outlet
perpetuating	being at home with two young children

Fig. 1.3 Predisposing, precipitating, and perpetuating factors in Mrs LM's depression.

THE PATIENT WITH ELEVATED MOOD

Mr EM is a 37-year-old married freelance writer who has been referred to psychiatric outpatients. He talks of periods of feeling depressed, during which he lacks energy, has difficulty in concentrating, eats too much, and has little or no sexual interest. Conversely, there are times when he feels 'euphoric' and has boundless energy, getting through large amounts of work. Initially the work is good, but he soon develops lofty ideas that he is a world expert in his field. He recalls volunteering to participate in elaborate and complicated writing schemes, only to find he is out of his depth when the euphoria has passed and then having to face the embarrassment of cobbling together a much truncated submission compared with what he had originally promised. During these periods (the last of which ended 6 weeks ago) he eats considerably less, requires little sleep, and has a greater sex drive—at times he has engaged in extramarital affairs. He has received speeding tickets, so his wife drives him to and from work during the episodes. Currently, Mr EM's mood is neither low nor elevated. He informs the psychiatrist that he spends about 6 months a year in this 'normal' phase; the periods of low and elevated mood each lasting an average of 3 months.

Psychopathology
Hypomanic and manic episodes
The symptoms and signs of hypomania and the more dramatic manic episodes are summarized in Fig. 1.4.

Manic episodes with psychotic features
More frequently than in depressive episodes, manic episodes may involve psychotic features, including disorders of thought-form, thought-content, and perception.

Disorders of thought-form
Disorders of thought-form may be seen in schizophrenia and are discussed in Chapter 5. They may also occur in association with manic episodes and in psychotic forms of unipolar depression. Circumstantiality, tangentiality, and flight of ideas typically occur in manic episodes with psychotic features, but loosening of associations, derailment, blocking, and neologisms (see Chapter 5) may also be observed.

Circumstantiality and tangentiality When a patient exhibits circumstantiality in speech, he or she may talk round and round a theme, with asides and diversions, before eventually getting to the intended point. In tangentiality, thought-disturbance is such that the patient deviates from the original topic and instead follows tangential thoughts, never returning to the intended point.

Flight of ideas Often seen in manic episodes, flight of ideas consists of a verbal stream of connected concepts. The link between each phrase or sentence may be through a pun or other play on words. The phenomenon is considered to be a psychotic feature when it is so extreme that the theme becomes impossible to understand or inaccessible to ordinary communications. Clang associations are illogical connections where words that rhyme or sound the same but are unrelated in meaning are used to form the link between one idea and the next. An example would be: 'What's happening in this case? . . . Cases have keys. . . . That's the key to the problem.'

Features of hypomanic and manic episodes		
Features	**Hypomanic episodes**	**Manic episodes**
mood	mildly elevated or irritable compared to usual	greatly elevated but may oscillate between mild elation and huge excitement, or person may appear grossly irritated or suspicious
duration	at least 4 consecutive days	at least 1 week
Symptoms & signs:	**(three or more of the following)**	**(three or more of the following, or four if mood is merely irritable)**
biological	increased energy/ restlessness decreased need for sleep increased sexual energy poor concentration	increased energy/restlessness decreased need for sleep marked sexual energy/sexual indiscretions distractibility or constant changes of plan
speech	increased talkativeness	increased talkativeness to extent of 'pressure of speech'
thought	—	flight of ideas (see text)
behaviour	increased sociability/ overfamiliarity irresponsibility or recklessness (e.g. mild overspending)	loss of social inhibitions leading to inappropriate behaviour foolhardy behaviour involving risks that are taken without insight (e.g. dangerous driving, gross overspending, foolish enterprises)
cognitive	—	inflated self-esteem/grandiosity

Fig. 1.4 Features of hypomanic and manic episodes.

Disorders of thought-content and perception

Disorders of thought-content (particularly delusions) and disorders of perception (hallucinations) occur in manic episodes that have reached the level of psychosis. The delusions are often related to the elevation in mood (i.e. are 'mood congruent'). Thus, typical delusions seen in manic episodes with psychotic features are those in which the patient believes they have special importance or unusual powers (grandiose delusions). Persecutory delusions may be mood congruent where the patient believes others are taking advantage of their apparent exalted status. Mood incongruent delusions are also seen. Delusions and hallucinations are discussed fully in Chapter 5.

Differential diagnosis

Bipolar affective disorder

In bipolar affective disorder, episodes both of elevated or irritable mood and increased energy and activity (hypomania or mania) and of low mood and decreased energy and activity (depression) may occur—hence the commonly used term 'manic–depressive illness'. Most of those who experience hypomanic or manic episodes also experience depressive periods, but a patient who has recurrent episodes of hypomania or mania without episodes of depressive symptoms is also classified as having bipolar affective disorder.

To make the ICD-10 diagnosis there must be either:
- At least one hypomanic or manic episode and at least one depressive episode.
- Two or more hypomanic or manic episodes.

It is usual to describe the nature of any current mood disturbance, specifying whether it is a depressive, hypomanic, or manic episode (e.g. 'bipolar affective disorder, current episode manic').

In the DSM-IV classification, the term 'bipolar I disorder' is applied to patients who reach mania in some or all of their episodes of elevated mood, and 'bipolar II disorder' to those whose periods of elevated mood never go beyond hypomania.

Manic or severe depressive episodes may further be described as being associated with psychotic features if, for example, hallucinations or delusions are present.

Cyclothymia

A diagnosis of cyclothymia requires:
- Two years of recurrent changes of mood involving many periods of low mood and depressive symptoms alternating with mild elation or hypomania. There may be periods of normal mood in between.
- The episodes are too short-lived or too mild to justify the diagnosis of bipolar affective disorder, but contain at least three depressive-like and three hypomanic-like symptoms.

Note that the diagnosis of cyclothymia can still be applied when previous manic or depressive episodes occurred prior to the period of 2 or more years of mood instability.

Depression

A mood disturbance involving only low mood (i.e. a unipolar rather than a bipolar illness) is categorized as a depressive disorder. Some patients who are recovering from a depressive episode appear to experience a transient period of mildly elevated mood. This can be explained by either ongoing antidepressant treatment or the sense of achievement at having escaped depression, and should not be considered indicative of a bipolar affective disorder.

Hypomanic or manic episodes secondary to organic disorders or to substances

In hypomanic or manic episodes induced by organic disorders or by substances, a general medical condition or other organic cause associated with mood elevation (Fig. 1.5) predates the development of mood disorder.

Personality disorders

Certain personality disorders may enter into the differential diagnosis (Fig. 1.6).

However, personality disorders involve stable and enduring behaviour patterns that do not wax and wane, unlike the more discrete manic or hypomanic episodes, and can usually be readily distinguished (see Chapter 8).

General medical and substance-related causes of hypomanic or manic episodes	
General medical conditions	**Substance-related**
lesions of frontal or temporal lobes, diencephalon or brainstem through neoplasia, trauma, infection	prolonged therapy with antidepressants amphetamines
thyroid disorders	hallucinogens
systemic lupus erythematosus	cocaine
renal failure	opiates
vitamin deficiencies	corticosteroids
	and very rarely, cimetidine, captopril, procyclidine

Fig. 1.5 General medical and substance-related causes of hypomanic or manic episodes.

Personality disorders having features similar to those found in hypomanic or manic episodes	
Personality disorder	**Features shared with hypomanic and manic episodes**
dissocial	disinhibition recklessness disregard for social norms
borderline	instability of mood recurrent changes of plan
histrionic	rapid mood change inappropriate behaviour continual search for excitement

Fig. 1.6 Personality disorders having features similar to those found in hypomanic or manic episodes.

Schizophrenia

In psychotic patients it is important to distinguish whether episodes are related to mania or to schizophrenia (see Chapter 5). Features suggestive of mania rather than schizophrenia are:

- Elevated mood with mood-congruent delusions (e.g. delusions of grandeur).
- Pressured speech.
- Hyperactivity and distractibility.
- Rapid onset.
- Presence of biological symptoms.

Delirium

For more information on delirium, see Chapter 10.

Discussion of vignette

What is the likely diagnosis?

Mr EM experiences periods of low mood in which he exhibits both biological (increased appetite, loss of sexual interest, poor concentration) and cognitive symptoms. These periods alternate with episodes in which his mood is elevated, again with corresponding biological features (reduced need for sleep and food, increased sexual interest) and during which he acts in an expansive manner and has an inflated self-image.

The pattern suggests that Mr EM has bipolar affective disorder, with the periods of low and elevated mood each lasting for about 3 months of the year, interspersed by periods of normal mood. The symptoms are presently in remission.

Cyclothymia can be ruled out as Mr EM's symptoms are too severe and last too long. He does not oscillate rapidly between highs and lows.

Other differential diagnoses that need to be considered for Mr EM include organic or substance-induced mood disorders.

Do Mr EM's periods of elevated mood constitute hypomanic or manic episodes?

Mr EM's elevation of mood during the episodes is out of keeping with his circumstances, and the episodes meet the criteria for mania. He exhibits grandiose ideas and an inflated self-esteem in volunteering to write articles that are beyond his means—and this has led to much embarrassment in the subsequent course of his work. He has behaved in a reckless manner behind the wheel of his car and, with his wife's co-operation, now avoids driving at these times. Extramarital affairs have occurred only in the periods of elevated mood and reflect both increased sexual drive and loss of social inhibition.

Using the ICD-10 classification we give Mr EM a diagnosis of bipolar affective disorder currently in remission, the latest episode being manic without psychotic symptoms. In the DSM-IV classification he would be considered to have bipolar I disorder, as opposed to bipolar II disorder in which episodes of elevated mood are no more than hypomanic.

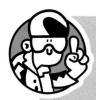

Mr EM has admitted to receiving speeding tickets. Since lack of insight is a feature of manic episodes, it is important to ask any patient who is suspected of having bipolar affective disorder whether they have had more serious trouble with the authorities. In manic episodes, patients may become disinhibited and contravene taboos, engaging in activities such as playing loud music which disturbs neighbours, or shoplifting.

2. Anxiety, Fear, and Avoidance

THE PATIENT WITH ANXIETY

Mr A, a 41 year old maintenance man, is referred to a consultant psychiatrist by his family doctor. He admits he has always been an 'anxious sort' and has been prone to periods when for no obvious reason he has felt under stress, with symptoms such as 'butterflies' in his stomach, sweating, and occasionally dizziness. During these periods he found it difficult to relax and felt constantly 'keyed-up' about the future, but all the symptoms would go away after a few days and the episodes caused him little inconvenience. However, he recalls taking a notable turn for the worse 4 months ago, when he began experiencing the same symptoms but in dramatic, devastating bursts that came on 'out of the blue' within 2 minutes. The attacks lasted 10–15 minutes and occurred two or three times a week. Mr A found these attacks extremely frightening: he was aware of his heart beating very strongly, which made him think he might die of a heart attack. At the height of the attacks he had difficulty catching his breath and was aware of a choking sensation. Mr A tells the psychiatrist that the worst thing about the attacks is that he never knows when they are going to happen. He has become so worried about having attacks outside his home that he has been on sick leave for the last 5 weeks and only ventures out in the company of his wife.

Psychopathology

Anxiety

Anxiety is the sense of apprehension at a perceived threat. The threat may be external and definite, as in specific phobias, or internal and less readily identifiable, as in generalized anxiety disorder and panic disorder.

Anxiety is not always pathological—it is perfectly appropriate to experience a degree of apprehension and anxiety when entering an oral examination, for example. Furthermore, in acutely dangerous situations, anxiety symptoms may provide a useful warning, alerting the body that swift action may be needed. Anxiety symptoms become psychiatric problems when they are chronic or recurrent and cause impairment to everyday life.

The ICD classification considers the numerous anxiety symptoms in five groups:

- Those produced by 'autonomic arousal'—palpitations, heart racing, tachycardia; sweating; trembling, shaking; dry mouth.
- Those involving the chest or abdomen—shortness of breath, difficulty in catching breath; choking sensation; chest pain or discomfort; nausea or abdominal distress (e.g. stomach churning).
- Those involving the mental state—feeling of being dizzy or about to faint; derealization (a sensation of things being 'unreal'); depersonalization (a sense of the self being distant and detached from the surroundings); fear of losing control, going mad, passing out, or dying.
- Other general symptoms—hot flushes or cold chills; numbness, tingling sensations; muscle tension, aches and pains; restlessness, inability to relax; feeling keyed-up, on edge, or mentally tense; sensation of a lump in the throat or difficulty in swallowing.

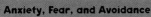

- Other non-specific symptoms—exaggerated response to minor surprises or being startled; poor concentration (e.g. mind going blank through worry); persistent irritability; difficulty getting to sleep through worrying.

Free-floating (or generalized) anxiety

As the name suggests, the onset of free-floating anxiety is not tied exclusively to one specific situation or known external threat. This is in contrast to anxiety symptoms that have a specific focus (Fig. 2.1), for instance in phobias (discussed later in this chapter), which represent a response to a definite, known, external threat. Instead, a collection of anxiety symptoms may appear in any situation and are persistent, lasting for hours, days, or even longer (Fig. 2.2). Typically, a patient may be generally worried about life situations such as work (e.g. job security or performance), relationships, or responsibilities.

Panic attacks

Panic attacks share many of the symptoms of free-floating or generalized anxiety. However, the key feature of the panic attack is that the symptoms are present for a discrete period only (see Fig. 2.2). Their onset is abrupt and they build up rapidly to their peak (normally within 10 minutes), during which time they may be extremely distressing and frightening for the patient. Often the presence of one symptom (e.g. palpitations) leads directly to another (e.g. fear of

having a heart attack)—this immediately increases the overall anxiety level and produces further symptoms (e.g. sweating, trembling) in a vicious cycle.

DSM-IV and ICD-10 list 13 and 14 symptoms, respectively, that are characteristic of panic attacks. The term 'panic attack' can only be applied if at least four of these symptoms are present; 'limited-symptom attacks' involve less than four symptoms.

The panic symptoms are:
- Palpitations, heart racing, tachycardia.
- Sweating.
- Trembling, shaking.
- Dry mouth.
- Shortness of breath, difficulty in catching breath.
- Choking sensation.
- Chest pain or discomfort.
- Nausea or abdominal distress.
- Dizziness, light-headedness, feeling unsteady or faint.
- Derealization.
- Depersonalization.
- Fear of losing control, going mad, passing out, or dying.
- Hot flushes or cold chills.
- Numbness, tingling.

Panic attacks occur in many anxiety disorders (Fig. 2.3), both in response to a specific external stimulus (e.g. a patient with arachnophobia has a panic attack on discovering a spider), and 'out of the blue' in the absence of any external stimulus, as occurs in panic disorder.

Diagnosis applicable when anxiety symptoms are focused on a specific factor	
Focus of anxiety and worry	**Probable diagnosis**
having panic attacks	panic disorder
being embarrassed in public or social situations	social phobia
having contact with a feared object or situation	specific phobia
having unwanted contact with the focus of obsessional thoughts (e.g. contamination)	obsessive–compulsive disorder
gaining weight	anorexia nervosa
having many physical complaints	somatization disorder
having one or more serious illnesses	hypochondriasis

Fig. 2.1 Diagnoses applicable when anxiety symptoms are focused on a specific factor.

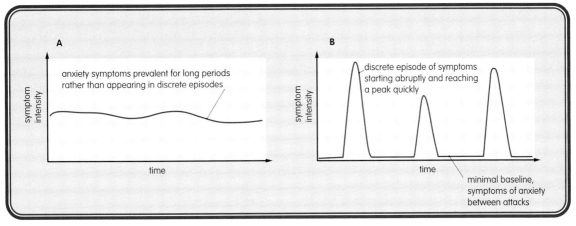

Fig. 2.2 Graphs showing free-floating (generalized) anxiety (A) compared with panic attacks (B).

Diagnoses applicable when panic attacks occur in specific circumstances	
Circumstance of attacks	**Diagnosis to consider**
in association with fear of a specific object or situation	specific phobia
in association with public speaking or social situations	social phobia
in association with obsessional thoughts or with a failure to carry out a compulsive act	obsessive–compulsive disorder
following a violent attack or other traumatic incident	post-traumatic stress disorder

Fig. 2.3 Diagnoses applicable when panic attacks occur in specific circumstances.

Anticipatory anxiety and agoraphobia

Some patients who experience spontaneous panic attacks are free of anxiety symptoms between attacks; others develop specific worries about having them again (i.e. anticipatory anxiety). Patients with agoraphobia are fearful of having panic attacks in situations where escape is embarrassing or difficult, and limit their travel and other activities accordingly.

Consider a man who suffers an unexpected panic attack while travelling on a bus. Feeling the need to escape to the fresh air outside, he shouts to the driver to stop and gets off in full view of the other passengers, much embarrassed as he trembles and gasps for breath while stumbling out. If he develops worries about having further attacks, he has anticipatory anxiety. If the thought of having another attack in an enclosed space like a bus makes him curtail his travels or insist on having an escort, he is likely to have agoraphobia.

Differential diagnosis

Generalized anxiety disorder

The key element of generalized anxiety disorder is long-standing free-floating anxiety. The diagnosis requires:

- Six months of apprehension and worry about everyday events and problems.
- At least four of the anxiety symptoms listed on page 13, at least one of which is from the autonomic arousal category.
- No evidence of an organic factor or substance causing the symptoms.

The DSM-IV criteria add that the patient must find the worry difficult to control, but limit the anxiety symptoms required to three from a core list of six.

Panic disorder

The key component in panic disorder is the discrete episode of fear or discomfort known as a panic attack.

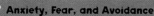
This diagnosis requires:
- Recurrent panic attacks with at least four of the panic symptoms listed on page 14.
- Attacks are unexpected rather than occurring in specific circumstances, and there is no evidence of an organic cause.
- Attacks start abruptly and reach a peak quickly.

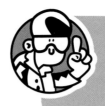

Remember that generalized anxiety disorder cannot be diagnosed unless the anxiety is predominantly free-floating.

While ICD-10 requires that at least one symptom in the attacks is from the autonomic arousal group, DSM-IV requires that at least one attack is followed by either persistent anticipatory anxiety, worry about its implications, or a significant behavioural change.

As the criteria for making a diagnosis of panic disorder are fairly complex, it is sometimes useful to ask a patient to keep a diary of panic attacks to see if they meet the criteria over a given period. The time of day, situation, and duration of attacks can be recorded and the presence or absence of each panic symptom can be indicated by ticks.

Panic disorder with agoraphobia

In panic disorder with agoraphobia, patients should not only meet the criteria for panic disorder but also display an avoidance or marked fear of any situation where, in the event of a panic attack, obtaining help might be difficult or escape might be hard or embarrassing. ICD-10 requires that there must have been anxiety symptoms when exposed to at least two of the following situations with subsequent avoidance:
- Crowds.
- Public places.
- Travelling alone.
- Travelling away from home.

Whilst agoraphobia usually results from the dread of having panic attacks in certain places or situations, it can occur without a diagnosis of panic disorder if the dreaded panic attacks have never occurred with sufficient frequency to meet the criteria. Agoraphobia can even be diagnosed without the occurrence of true panic attacks if only two or three anxiety symptoms, such as dizziness or trembling, are experienced and their onset subsequently feared. These symptoms would be too few in number to be considered a panic attack,

but might still provoke sufficient fear to cause avoidance of the situation in which they were experienced.

Depression and other affective disorders
See Chapter 1 for more information.

Anxiety symptoms often occur together with symptoms of depressive or bipolar affective disorders. To make a diagnosis, it is essential to decide which symptoms came first or were predominant and which were secondary to the main diagnosis. If depression and an anxiety disorder appear to have developed independently and distinctly, rather than one being secondary to the other, both diagnoses are applied.

Anxiety related to general medical conditions or substances
An important differential that always needs to be ruled out before diagnosing an anxiety disorder is the possibility that symptoms are a direct consequence of a general medical condition or are due to side effects of, intoxication with, or withdrawal from, ingested substances (Fig. 2.4).

Other psychiatric disorders
When anxiety symptoms are directly associated with any of the specific objects, situations, symptoms, or illnesses listed in Fig. 2.1, rather than being free-floating, then the adjacent disorder should be diagnosed.

Panic attacks may also occur in several other anxiety disorders, but, unlike in panic disorder, where some or all of the attacks are spontaneous, there is a predictable circumstance in which all attacks occur (see Fig. 2.3).

General medical conditions and substances that may be associated with anxiety			
General medical conditions	**Substances**		
	intoxication	**side effects of prescribed drugs**	**withdrawal**
hyperthyroidism temporal lobe epilepsy phaeochromocytoma hypoglycaemia Cushing's disease congestive cardiac failure pulmonary embolism chronic obstructive airways disease vitamin deficiencies malignancies cerebral trauma	alcohol amphetamines caffeine cannabis cocaine hallucinogens inhalants phencycclidene	analgesics anticholinergics antihistamines antidepressants (e.g. SSRIs in first 2 weeks of use) antipsychotics corticosteroids insulin lithium oral contraceptives sympathomimetics thyroid hormone	alcohol caffeine cocaine benzodiazepines nicotine other sedatives and hypnotics
(N.B. exposure to toxins such as mercury, organophosphates, petrol fumes, or carbon monoxide may also cause anxiety)			

Fig. 2.4 General medical conditions and substances that may be associated with anxiety. (SSRI, selective serotonin reuptake inhibitors.)

Discussion of vignette

How would you describe Mr A's symptoms up to 4 months ago?
The symptoms Mr A was experiencing prior to the change 4 months ago are suggestive of free-floating anxiety. They comprised a typical selection of anxiety symptoms and appeared not to be restricted to any particular circumstance or situation, simply reflecting general concerns in his life. They came episodically without a sudden onset and faded away gradually. Had Mr A been sufficiently troubled by these symptoms to seek psychiatric help at that stage, it is likely that he would have been given a diagnosis of generalized anxiety disorder.

What is Mr A's current diagnosis?
The pattern of Mr A's symptoms changed dramatically 4 months ago. His anxiety began to occur in discrete attacks that came on suddenly, reached a peak quickly, and lasted a relatively short time. At least four of the panic symptoms were present during the attacks, thus fulfilling the criteria for panic attacks. As attacks have occurred at the rate of four or more in 4 weeks, and some or all of them have been spontaneous rather than as a consequence of

exposure to a particular situation or circumstance, the primary diagnosis for Mr A is now panic disorder.

Note that between attacks Mr A's panic symptoms remit completely and his only symptoms are those of 'anticipatory anxiety' about having further attacks. The anticipatory anxiety has led to Mr A avoiding going out to work or even leaving the house unaccompanied—he therefore may be developing an additional diagnosis of agoraphobia.

What questions would rule out other differentials?
Closer questioning could reveal that Mr A's symptoms were predominantly due to exposure to a particular feared stimulus or circumstance, such as thunderstorms or seeing Alsatian dogs, rather than occurring entirely unexpectedly—if so, a specific phobia would be a more appropriate diagnosis. Experience of traumatic stress or of obsessional thoughts and compulsive acts should also be elicited. We would also wish to look for evidence of medical or substance-related causes.

When enquiring about a mood disorder, we would be particularly interested in the time of onset, to ascertain which came first—depression may have developed independently of, or secondarily to, the panic disorder.

THE PATIENT WITH FEAR OR AVOIDANCE

> Miss FA is 24 years old and has worked for a marketing company since leaving school. She has carried out her duties with efficiency and last year earned a well-deserved promotion to a post with greater responsibility. Unfortunately, the new job involved presenting sales figures to her colleagues in a monthly meeting. Miss FA had no previous experience of public speaking and became very fearful of attending the first meeting. Even thinking about making the presentation made her tremble and blush and caused her stomach to churn and her heart to beat faster. She resolved to stand up and deliver as short a report as possible. However, she recalls that when introduced she was trembling, feeling breathless, and perspiring profusely, and she grabbed the lectern tightly for fear of falling over or collapsing. The chairman realized she was in some distress and read out the figures himself, asking Miss FA a simple question to which she replied 'That's right', and then excused her. Miss FA continued to cope well with every other aspect of the job but was acutely fearful of the next meeting. She arranged a fortnight's holiday to avoid the second presentation and decided to consult her family doctor during this time.

Psychopathology
Fear and phobias
A phobic patient may exhibit any or all of the anxiety symptoms listed on page 13 and may also experience panic attacks. However, the symptoms occur in direct response to an external stimulus, usually a well-defined situation that most people would not normally consider dangerous. The symptoms are evoked not only by encountering the feared situation or object but also by mere contemplation of such.

Avoidance
A person who has a phobia will often aim to avoid the feared stimulus. In some phobias (e.g. fear of travelling in lifts) this may be relatively easy (unless the sufferer lives or works on the top floor of a tower block) and can be achieved without excessive disruption to the person's lifestyle.

In some cases, however, the feared object or situation can be avoided only by withdrawing from some facets of usual function, e.g. a person who develops a fear of thunderstorms may choose to stay at home, defaulting on work or social commitments, on a day when storms are forecast.

We have already seen that avoidance is prevalent in agoraphobia, where concerns about the implications of having a panic attack in a public place where escape could be difficult makes the patient avoid such places. In severe cases, avoidance dominates, with the patient staying at home unless escorted.

Differential diagnosis
Social phobia
A patient with social phobia has:
- Fear of being the focus of attention or of acting in a way that causes self-humiliation, or avoidance of situations like public speaking or meetings where one of these fears may be met.
- At least two of the anxiety symptoms listed on page 13, as well as one symptom out of blushing, shaking, and fear of being sick, micturition, or defecation.
- Symptoms brought on only by entering or contemplating these situations.
- Significant emotional distress due to the symptoms or the avoidance.

Specific phobia

In specific phobia the patient has:

- Fear of exposure to an object or situation (other than those covered in social phobia and agoraphobia), or marked avoidance of the object or situation.
- At least two of the anxiety symptoms listed on page 13.
- Symptoms brought on only by exposure to, or contemplation of, the object or situation.
- Significant emotional distress due to the symptoms or the avoidance.

Examples of objects or situations that may be associated with specific phobias are:

- Spiders.
- Dogs.
- Mice.
- Needles (or having to give a blood sample).
- Heights.
- Flying.

Other differential diagnoses

Other differentials comprise:

- Agoraphobia, generalized anxiety disorder, and panic disorder (see pages 15–16).
- Obsessive–compulsive disorder (see Chapter 3).
- Post-traumatic stress disorder and adjustment reactions (see Chapter 4).
- Depressive disorders (see Chapter 1).

Discussion of vignette

What is Miss FA's likely diagnosis?

Like Mr A in the previous section, Miss FA has exhibited multiple symptoms, in her case including tremor, blushing, palpitations, and abdominal distress.

Where she differs markedly from Mr A, however, is that her symptoms are clearly and demonstrably associated with one particular situation: the monthly presentation. Note that the symptoms first occur merely on contemplation of having to present. Then, when Miss FA is about to be meet the object of her fear—having to stand up and present the figures to the audience of her colleagues—she experiences a dramatic surge of symptoms.

This crescendo has some characteristics of a panic attack: the symptoms develop quickly and peak rapidly, with excessive trembling and palpitations that make

Miss FA feel she is going to collapse and lose control. In panic disorder, such attacks might come on without an obvious provoking stimulus, but here the attack is a consequence of being placed in a situation that is perceived as threatening.

The direct association of the symptoms with thinking about or experiencing the feared situation means that neither generalized anxiety disorder nor panic disorder are appropriate diagnoses, and it is likely that Miss FA's symptoms are due to social phobia. Her fear of speaking in public—a situation in which she is briefly the focus of attention and subject to the scrutiny of her colleagues—is responsible for her symptoms, which are similar to those encountered in free-floating anxiety. They include blushing and shaking, which are particularly common in social phobia.

Many people are genuinely afraid of having to speak in a public gathering; however, Miss FA feels that her symptoms are particularly excessive, and the problem has caused her sufficient distress that she has sought medical assistance. She is also beginning to exhibit avoidance of the feared situation, deliberately timing her holiday to miss the next meeting.

What other differential diagnoses could be considered?

There is no evidence that Miss FA suffers from specific phobias (e.g. to animals, insects, or heights), but it would be worth asking about this in case a specific phobia is also present. Agoraphobia is not an appropriate diagnosis as she is capable of going out and performing satisfactorily in her work for the rest of the month.

Adjustment reaction (see Chapter 4) is worth considering, as she may be having difficulty adjusting to the demands of her new promotion; however, the symptoms are overwhelmingly specific to contemplation of, or exposure to, public speaking where she is the focus of attention, and she copes well with all the other demands of the new job. Therefore, social phobia is the more likely diagnosis.

As with Mr A, a history of depressive symptoms, traumatic events, and obsessional thoughts should be elicited to establish whether a primary or co-morbid depressive disorder, post-traumatic stress disorder, or obsessive–compulsive disorder is present.

3. Obsessionality and Compulsiveness

THE PATIENT WHO EXHIBITS OBSESSIONALITY AND COMPULSIVENESS

Mr OC is 36 and lives on his own. He complains of recurrent thoughts about the dangers of contamination of his skin by dirt and dust from household objects. The only way he can escape from such thoughts and the worry they engender is to wash his hands regularly—recently up to 10 times in an hour. He is also repeatedly concerned that his food must be free from any chance of contamination and has developed an elaborate procedure for preparing simple meals which takes nearly 3 hours. He is extremely frustrated by the amount of time used for both hand washing and food preparation, and sees this as a senseless waste. However, despite genuine effort, he is unable to resist either these activities or the constant thoughts about dirt and contamination. He is frequently low in mood and often exhibits anxiety. He tells you he has lost a stone in weight over the last 6 months and you notice that his palms are red and excoriated.

Psychopathology

Obsessions and compulsions

Obsessions are recurrent and persistent ideas, impulses, or images that are experienced as intrusive and inappropriate and cause marked anxiety and distress. The patient recognizes them as his or her own thoughts, and may try to resist, but may find them impossible to remove. In adults the most common obsessions involve:

- Thoughts of contamination.
- Pathological doubt (e.g. of whether simple tasks have been properly completed).
- Thoughts of having physical (somatic) symptoms.
- Symmetry (e.g. of household articles).
- Aggressive thoughts.

Compulsions are recurrent and persistent behaviours or mental acts undertaken to prevent or reduce anxiety or distress, usually through the belief that they will prevent a dreaded event from occurring. They do not produce pleasure or gratification, nor do the tasks they involve bring useful results. However, if they are resisted, the level of anxiety may increase. The most commonly reported compulsions are:

- Checking.
- Washing.
- Counting.
- Needing to ask questions or make confessions.
- Creating symmetry and order.
- Needing to be precise.

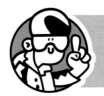

It is important to memorize the definitions of obsessions and compulsions.

Obsessions and compulsions are often inextricably linked, as the desire to resist an obsessional thought produces a compulsive act (Fig. 3.1).

Obsessions and compulsions have a number of features in common. For example:

- The ideas or impulses are recurrent.
- They are a product of the patient's own mind (unlike passivity phenomena—see Chapter 5).
- They are accompanied by feelings of dread.
- The sufferer tries to fight them off.

Although attempts to resist may dwindle in time, the patient always remains aware that both the obsessional thoughts and the compulsive acts are absurd.

Overvalued ideas

An overvalued idea is an isolated belief which the person returns to recurrently. It is not an obsession and its content is not delusional, but it may preoccupy the individual to such an extent that it dominates their life for several years and has an effect on their actions. Events during the person's life may be directly connected with the belief and make the preoccupation understandable. For instance, a person whose parents both died of heart attacks may become preoccupied with the idea that heart disease is infectious.

Differential diagnosis

Obsessive–compulsive disorder

The diagnosis of obsessive–compulsive disorder requires that:

- Repetitive and unpleasant obsessions or compulsions occur on most days for at least 2 weeks.

- They are acknowledged to originate from the patient's own mind.
- At least one obsession or compulsion is seen as excessive or unreasonable.
- Resistance is (or has been) attempted and at least one obsession or compulsion is resisted unsuccessfully.

Obsessions and compulsions impair functioning (usually by wasting time) and are not actually pleasurable, although they may relieve anxiety.

Other anxiety disorders

The anxiety produced by obsessive–compulsive disorder is easily differentiated from that seen in phobias because the provoking stimulus comes from within the patient's mind rather than being an external object or situation. Generalized anxiety disorder and panic disorder can be ruled out once it is established that anxiety symptoms or panic attacks are associated with obsessional thoughts or compulsive acts rather than being free-floating or unpredictable (see Figs 2.1 and 2.3).

Depression (with obsessional thoughts)

Over two-thirds of patients with obsessive–compulsive disorder experience major depression during their lives. Occasionally, a person who has depression may appear to be 'obsessed' with unpleasant circumstances and unhappy events. Remember that such thoughts are a mood-congruent aspect of depression which can lead on to mood-congruent delusions of failure, worthlessness, or emptiness. Such thoughts lack the definitive characteristics of obsessions and are not associated with compulsive acts.

Examples of closely linked obsessions and compulsions	
Obsession	**Compulsion**
contamination	hand-washing avoidance of dust, germs or urine
doubt (e.g. have I switched the cooker off?)	repeated checking of the object of doubt
need for symmetry	compulsive slowness in maintaining symmetry

Fig. 3.1 Examples of closely linked obsessions and compulsions.

Schizophrenia

It may be sometimes necessary to rule out the presence of psychotic phenomena in a patient with obsessions or compulsions. For instance, a regular feature in schizophrenia is thought-insertion, where the patient believes thoughts are entering their head from some external source such as a transmitter or the television. By contrast, in obsessive–compulsive disorder, the obsessions are recognized by the sufferer as a product of their own mind and cannot be considered as delusional. Further features that point towards obsessive–compulsive disorder are the absence of other schizophrenic symptoms, the symptoms being less bizarre, and the retention of insight.

Obsessive–compulsive (anankastic) personality disorder

This personality disorder (see Chapter 8) involves an enduring behaviour pattern of features such as rigidity, doubt, perfectionism, and pedantry, but there are no true obsessions or compulsions.

Eating disorders

In anorexia nervosa (see Chapter 10), a distortion of body image may be reflected by a preoccupation with fatness and a strong desire to lose weight. Although the weight loss is sometimes described as compulsive, obsessive–compulsive disorder cannot generally be diagnosed. In the anorexic patient, the thoughts and actions may not be recognized as excessive or unreasonable and are not resisted, nor do the thoughts necessarily provoke, or the actions reduce, distress.

Gilles de la Tourette's syndrome

There is sometimes diagnostic confusion between obsessive–compulsive disorder and the tic disorder Gilles de la Tourette's syndrome: both disorders affect young people, two-thirds of obsessive–compulsive disorder cases having onset before the age of 25 years and Gilles de la Tourette's syndrome by definition occurring before the age of 18 years. As many as 90% of patients with this syndrome, in which motor and vocal tics occur, frequently appear to display compulsive acts.

Temporal lobe epilepsy

Temporal lobe epilepsy may also be confused for obsessive–compulsive disorder: the complex partial seizures can produce disturbances of speech and thought, and repetitive movements or repeated behaviours. Transient impairment of consciousness and the presence of an aura are features that would point towards this diagnosis.

Discussion of vignette

What is Mr OC's likely diagnosis?

It is likely that Mr OC fulfils the criteria for a diagnosis of obsessive–compulsive disorder. His thoughts about contamination are recurrent and persistent and generate anxiety—they therefore constitute obsessional thoughts. His worries are certainly intrusive and inappropriate rather than simply being excessive concerns about real-life problems. He is driven to wash his hands repeatedly in order to neutralize this worry. There is no pleasure in the hand-washing activity—it is undertaken only to contain his worries about the spread of contamination. However, in spite of trying to resist it and seeing the whole thing as senseless, he has to carry on. The hand washing is excessive compared with that really necessary to prevent infections, and given these features, it fulfils the criteria as being a compulsive act.

Obsession with contamination and compulsive hand washing is one of the most commonly observed patterns in obsessive–compulsive disorder. The excoriation of Mr OC's palms is a consequence of the excessive hand washing and may require the attention of a dermatologist.

What other diagnoses could be considered?

The symptoms are too severe and have developed too late in life for a diagnosis of anankastic personality disorder to be appropriate. Individuals

Having an obsessive–compulsive personality disorder predisposes to depressive disorders more than to the development of obsessive–compulsive disorder.

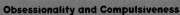

with this personality disorder do not have the same degree of functional impairment as Mr OC, and although their perfectionism can cause dysfunction and distress, importantly they do not have true obsessions or compulsions.

It is not surprising that Mr OC suffers episodes of low mood when we remember how frustrated he feels at wasting so much time in activities he sees as senseless.

Clearly this low mood is secondary to his obsessive–compulsive symptoms and does not justify a further diagnosis of 'depressive episode'.

The weight loss is a consequence of Mr OC's failure to eat adequately—the amount of time he has to invest in the compulsive acts is a great disincentive to do any cooking. It is not a consequence of depression nor of an eating disorder.

4. Reaction to Stress or to a Traumatic Event

THE PATIENT REACTING TO STRESS OR TO A TRAUMATIC EVENT

Mrs ST, aged 50, attends a day centre run by the local psychiatric services. She was perfectly well until 2 months ago, working as an office cleaner. She usually travelled home from work by bus. One dark evening she was waiting alone in the shelter when two youths approached. They pushed her violently to the ground, injuring her wrist, and made off with her handbag before the bus arrived. She felt low in mood for a few days after the assault, but attempted to carry on with her job. Unfortunately, she soon began to experience flashbacks to the incident, especially on seeing young people in small groups. She became hypervigilant and was careful to avoid bus-stops, as seeing them also made her think of the attack, and she had to arrange for her husband to pick her up in his car. She was generally irritable and reported feeling numb and anxious. After 4 weeks of trying to continue at work, she could no longer concentrate properly on the job. She told her supervisor the whole story and was granted sick leave. With the flashbacks continuing, her family doctor arranged for her to be seen in the day centre.

Psychopathology

Stress
Stress is a general term for the experience of any life event to which the individual cannot adequately respond. It is a person's response to an inappropriate level of pressure and involves a mismatch between their perceived or actual ability and the demands of the situation. Work or exam pressures are common stressors, and events such as divorce or job loss may produce more severe stress.

Traumatic stress
A traumatic stressor has the more specific ingredient of being extremely threatening, with the real possibility of danger to 'life and limb'. Exposure to military combat, natural or man-made disasters, fatal or near-fatal accidents, and violent or potentially violent personal attacks fall into this category.

Adjustment
Sometimes, anxiety symptoms or features typical of depression occur after a change in circumstances that has forced an individual to make adjustments in their life rather than after an acutely traumatic event. Examples include moving to a new area or foreign country, becoming a parent, and being promoted (or failing to achieve an expected promotion), or taking on new responsibilities.

Flashbacks
Patients who experience flashbacks have recurrent intrusive memories of an event, in particular one that was traumatic or caused severe stress.

Bereavement and the grieving process
Bereavement is a well-characterized traumatic event. When a person loses a spouse, close relative or friend,

25

a grieving process or bereavement reaction is initiated (Fig. 4.1).

Although most people who experience bereavement are sufficiently low in mood to meet the criteria for a depressive episode at some point following their loss, normal bereavement reactions are not pathological and no psychiatric diagnosis is made in these circumstances. However, the grieving process sometimes stalls at the denial, anger, or grief stage, and the person fails to pass on to resolution. Bereavement reactions are considered abnormal and may be diagnosed as a form of adjustment disorder when they last for more than 6 months or involve unusually pronounced symptoms.

Dissociation
Dissociation is a loss of control of bodily function arising from a failure to integrate past memories with current sensations and identity. Amnesia, fugue, or stupor (see Fig. 4.1) can be provoked by stressful events or emotional conflicts through this dissociative process.

Differential diagnosis
Acute stress reaction
The diagnosis of acute stress reaction requires:
- Exposure to a 'stressor' event or situation involving exceptional physical or mental stress.
- The appearance of anxiety symptoms within 1 hour of the event or situation.

Other symptoms may also be present. These include:
- Social withdrawal.
- Narrowed field of attention.
- Disorientation.
- Despair or hopelessness.
- Inappropriate overactivity.
- Excessive grief.

ICD-10 considers episodes to be severe if four of these symptoms are present, or moderate if two occur.

Post-traumatic stress disorder
For a diagnosis of post-traumatic stress disorder, there must be exposure to a 'stressor' event or situation that is highly threatening or catastrophic.

All of the following must subsequently develop (usually within 6 months, but in exceptional cases, over a longer period):

- Re-living of the event in flashbacks, vivid memories, or dreams, or distress caused by exposure to cues associated with the stressor.
- Onset of avoidance of circumstances associated with or resembling the stressor.
- Partial or complete amnesia of exposure to the stressor, or persistent symptoms of increased psychological sensitivity and arousal (including two of the following: difficulty falling or staying asleep, irritability or angry outbursts, poor concentration, hypervigilance, exaggerated startle response).

Adjustment disorder
In adjustment reactions, patients present with symptoms normally associated with depression (e.g. low mood, poor appetite, poor sleep), but short of psychotic features such as delusions and hallucinations, or with symptoms of anxiety (e.g. tremor, sweating, palpitations).

The symptoms are directly related to a change in life requiring adaptation, which must occur less than 1 month before symptom onset.

Abnormal bereavement reaction
An abnormal reaction to bereavement (in which the grieving process has lasted more than 6 months or contains unusually pronounced symptoms of denial, anger, or grief) is a form of adjustment disorder.

Dissociative (conversion) disorders
Dissociative disorders (Fig. 4.2) are also thought to occur in response to stressful events. To diagnose one of these disorders there must be convincing evidence of a chronological association between the onset of the symptoms and stressful events or problems. In addition, there must be no evidence of a physical disorder that would explain the symptoms.

Acute and transient psychotic disorders
These disorders are considered in Chapter 5. Onset may be precipitated by acute stress, but, unlike the disorders considered above, they include acute onset of delusions, hallucinations, or incoherent speech.

Other differential diagnoses
Other differentials comprise:
- Generalized anxiety disorder, panic disorder, and phobias (see Chapter 2).
- Depressive disorders (see Chapter 1).

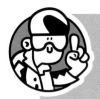

ICD-10 allows the dissociative disorders to be given the alternative name of 'conversion disorders', but watch out—the American DSM-IV classification reserves the term 'conversion disorder' for a specific syndrome where one or more neurological symptoms are caused by psychological stressors (see Chapter 9).

Discussion of vignette
What features suggest the likely diagnosis of post-traumatic stress disorder?

Mrs ST suffered a stressful and traumatic event—the violent attack, injury, and loss of her property, which most people would consider a threatening experience. After a characteristic delay (in some cases of post-traumatic stress disorder, this delay may be up to 6 months or much longer), she began to re-live the experience through flashbacks, and these were worse when she was exposed to circumstances resembling the event—the approach of youths or seeing bus shelters. The experience has engendered avoidance—she has modified her arrangements so that she no longer travels by bus. She has become irritable and hypervigilant and has difficulty in concentrating.

Stages of a normal bereavement reaction	
Stages of bereavement	**Description of stage**
denial	disbelief of the news of the death: 'It can't be true'
anger	'How unfair that they should die' or 'How could they die and leave me to cope?'
grief	sadness, weepiness and other symptoms seen in depression such as poor sleep, appetite loss and poor concentration
resolution	gradual acceptance of loss

Fig. 4.1 Stages of a normal bereavement reaction.

Characteristics of dissociative disorders	
Dissociative disorder	**Characteristics**
dissociative amnesia	periods of memory loss, usually of stressful or traumatic events memory loss is partial but more significant than mere forgetfulness
dissociative fugue	more complex than dissociative amnesia, fugues involve periods of spontaneous but apparently organized travel. The person appears organized but may lose all recall of their journey after returning
dissociative stupor	a more dramatic condition in which voluntary movement, speech and normal responsiveness to external stimuli (light, noise, touch) are much reduced. May be a feature of a severe acute stress reaction

Fig. 4.2 Characteristics of dissociative disorders.

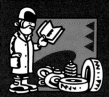

5. Delusions and Hallucinations

Mr DH, aged 23, was assessed by the on-call GP because of concerns about his behaviour. Over the last 6 months he had become increasingly reclusive, spending more time in his flat and refusing to answer the door. He had terminated his part-time work and had stopped seeing his friends. When he agreed to see the GP, he disclosed that government scientists had started to perform experiments on him over the last year. These involved the insertion of an electrode into his brain which was sensitive to gamma rays—such rays would be directly transmitted to him in order for him to obey their commands, thus proving telepathy was possible. The rays were able to hypnotize him and introduce a series of unpleasant images into his mind. He first became aware of the scientists' actions when he overheard someone in a pub conversing about the dangers of nuclear experiments. Recently, Mr DH had heard the scientists discussing him on the television and radio whenever they were switched on. When the GP suggested there might be an alternative explanation for these experiences, Mr DH became increasingly irate, accusing all doctors and scientists of working together.

Psychopathology

The vignette illustrates a disturbed and distorted view of reality, involving abnormalities of thought-content and perception, with deterioration of personal functioning. This chapter will concentrate on the most distinctive symptoms of psychosis: delusions and hallucinations.

Delusions

Definition

A delusion is defined as an unshakeable false belief or idea, held with subjective certainty on inadequate grounds, which is out of keeping with that person's social or cultural background.

It follows from this definition that the following criteria must be met to establish an idea as delusional:

- Subjective certainty—a patient cannot complain of a delusion, it can only be diagnosed by an observer, because the belief is recognized as the patient's own (i.e. it is indistinguishable from their other true

beliefs). The belief should be held without any doubt and should not be amenable to persuasion.

- Held on illogical grounds—the thought processes leading to an abnormal belief must be shown to be illogical. For example, one man might believe his wife was being unfaithful to him because she returned from work later than usual; another may have the same belief just because a new government has been elected. While the former may be seen as a plausible argument, the latter is totally implausible.
- The belief is false—delusions are usually bizarre and improbable from the outset. This may be less obvious where there are themes of persecution or jealousy (as in the case above). In rare cases the delusional idea is true, but this is coincidental; at the heart of a delusion is the illogical reasoning.
- It is out of keeping with that person's background—it is important to establish that the belief is not one likely to be held by that person's subcultural group.

For example, a belief in the imminent second coming of Christ may be appropriate for a member of a certain religious cult, but not for a formerly atheist, middle-aged businessman.

Delusions are classified according to their form and content.

Form

Secondary

Secondary delusions occur as a consequence of existing psychopathology and are therefore understandable to some extent; for example, the severely depressed patient who believes his bowels are rotting away inside his body, or the manic patient who develops a belief he is the second son of God.

Primary

A primary or autochthonous delusion is a delusional idea that occurs suddenly and unexpectedly, with no precipitating psychopathology.

Three specific types of primary delusional experiences are described:

- Delusional perception—a false meaning is attributed to a normal perception, e.g. a person believes he is the target of the CIA because his post went to the wrong address one morning.
- Delusional memory—a false meaning is attributed to a memory of an event that occurred before the patient's illness, e.g. a person believes he is the target of the CIA because of anaesthetic complications during a childhood operation. This differs from delusional retrospective falsifications, where there is backdating of delusional ideas prior to that person's illness, e.g. the patient says they were always subject to CIA surveillance, and that the CIA caused the anaesthetic complications.
- Delusional mood—the patient has a sense that the outside world has altered, often in a sinister, threatening way, with a feeling of anxiety or foreboding for the future. Delusional mood often precedes fully formed delusional ideas; the affective component of this state is known as perplexity.

Secondary delusions may develop from each of these primary forms. Complex, interrelated delusions are referred to as systematized delusions.

Content

Many types are described (Fig 5.1).

'Paranoid' delusions

This is a collective term denoting those delusions that are self-referent to the patient, i.e. delusions of reference, persecution, jealousy, and religion.

Partial delusions

Partial delusions are ideas that were previously held with delusional intensity but which are now held with less conviction. They are encountered frequently during recovery from, or after treatment of, a mental illness.

Overvalued ideas

Overvalued ideas are strongly held, preoccupying beliefs which are understandable in the context of a person's life history, social and cultural background, and current life circumstances.

It is vital to separate overvalued ideas from delusions. Both contain a subjective sense of conviction and may appear bizarre or incomprehensible to the observer; often they cause a similar degree of suffering. However, overvalued ideas do not involve a clear abnormality of reasoning. They may be viewed as pathological, e.g. abnormal ideas of body image associated with eating disorders (see Chapter 10), or non-pathological, e.g. the 'eccentric' scientist who adheres to theories not accepted by the mainstream. They are most difficult to distinguish from secondary delusions where ideas can be understood in respect to existing psychopathology. In severe depression, a patient might blame himself for his recent redundancy, relecting overvalued ideas of guilt: if he blamed himself for nation-wide redunancies, this might reflect delusional ideas of guilt. A comparison of delusions, obsessions, and overvalued ideas is shown in Fig. 5.2.

Hallucinations

Abnormalities of sensory perception are a common finding in mental illness. Of greatest diagnostic significance is the hallucination.

Definition

A hallucination is defined as an involuntary false perception occurring in the absence of an external stimulus but which exhibits the quality of a true percept.

Classification of delusions by their content	
Classification	**Content**
delusions of persecution	these are the commonest type encountered, they involve a belief that the patient is in some way being harmed or interfered with by another agency
delusions of reference	these concern a belief that certain objects, people or events have a personal significance to the patient, for example, a patient believes a recent disaster seen on TV proves he is about to die; similarly, a patient believes the doctor's tie was worn in recognition of his religious powers
grandiose delusions	here the patient has an exaggerated sense of his own abilities or importance, for example, a patient believes he is on a special mission to save mankind
religious delusions	these are common, for example, a patient believes he was the Antichrist. It is particularly important that such beliefs are shown to be distinct from existing subcultural religious beliefs
delusions of love	here the patient believes another person is in love with her. In one form, usually affecting women, the person believes a person of higher status (e.g. TV celebrity) and usually quite inaccessible, is in love with her (de Clerambault's syndrome)
delusions of jealousy	these patients believe their partner is being unfaithful
delusions of misidentification	two forms are notable: • Capgras delusion: the patient believes someone close to him has been replaced by a double even though their appearance is the same • Fregoli delusion: the patient identifies a person known to him in other people he meets, even though the appearances are dissimilar
nihilistic delusions	the patient negates some part of himself or the outside world to the extent that they do not exist, for example, a belief part of their body is dying or rotting; or a belief the world is about to end
delusions of guilt or unworthiness	common in depression, e.g. patient believes he is to blame for a global catastrophe
hypochondriacal delusions	these are concerned with the presence of illness despite all evidence to the contrary
delusions of infestation	the patient believes their body is infested with other organisms, e.g. spiders, often this is in association with hallucinations of bodily sensation; this symptom is also known as Ekbom's syndrome
delusions of control	also known as Passivity or Made experiences, the patient believes his actions, impulses and emotions are controlled by an external agency, for example, a patient believes that he was made to drive through red traffic lights by demons
delusions of the control of thought: • thought insertion • thought withdrawal • thought broadcast	similar to above, the patient believes their thoughts are not their own and controlled by external agencies: • the patient experiences alien thoughts implanted by an external agency • the patient experiences thoughts being extracted from their mind; this is often the delusional explanation for thought blocking • the patient believes others are aware of, or can hear, his own thoughts

Fig. 5.1 Classification of delusions by their content.

Several points arise from this definition:
- They are experienced as sensations via any one of the sense organs—therefore they should be distinguished from ideas, images, or fantasy which originate in the patient's own mind.
- They occur without an external stimulus—therefore they are not distortions of an existing sensory stimulus.
- They appear to the patient as real—as with delusions, they are diagnosed by the observer, and the patient often has no insight into their abnormal experience.

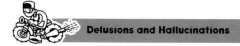

Comparison of delusions, obsessions, and overvalued ideas			
	Delusion	**Obsession**	**Overvalued idea**
preoccupying belief/thought	+/−	+	+/−
recognized as patient's own thought	+/− (1)	+	+
resisted by patient	−	+	−
unshakeable belief	+	−	+/−
understandable in terms of patient's background/personality/circumstances	−	−	+
indicate psychiatric disorder	+	+	+/−

(1)=may involve experiences of thought alienation, e.g. thought insertion

Fig. 5.2 Comparison of delusions, obsessions, and overvalued ideas.

Auditory hallucinations

Auditory hallucinations are by far the most common type of hallucination encountered in clinical psychiatry and can take a variety of forms.

Elementary hallucination

Elementary hallucinations are perceived as simple noises, e.g. whistles, claps, or single words.

Complex hallucination

Complex hallucinations are perceived as phrases, sentences, or even whole conversations. This form can be further subdivided as follows:

- First person—the patient is able to hear their own thoughts spoken aloud, or hears a voice anticipating or echoing their own thoughts.
- Second person—the patient hears a voice or voices talking directly to them. The content is highly variable: it may be complimentary or accusatory, or it may be commanding the patient to do something.
- Third person—the patient hears two or more voices talking to each other, often making reference to the patient. As well as discussing the patient, they may also give a running commentary on the patient's thoughts or actions.

Visual hallucinations

Visual hallucinations are encountered less frequently in clinical psychiatry and are usually associated with organic disorders. Again, they may appear in elementary (e.g. wavy lines, light flashes) or complex (e.g. animals, human figures) forms.

Autoscopic hallucination

An autoscopic hallucination is the experience of seeing one's own body projected into external space. It differs from a Capgras delusion, where the original perception is normal.

Charles Bonnet syndrome

In Charles Bonnet syndrome, vivid, complex visual hallucinations occur in the presence of existing loss of central or peripheral vision.

Hallucinations of bodily sensation

Hallucinations of bodily sensation are often the most difficult to establish objectively—frequently, a patient's description of such is complicated by a delusion, especially one of infestation or control.

Tactile (haptic) hallucination

Tactile hallucination describes sensations on or just below the skin, e.g. being touched, pricked, pinched, or feeling insects crawling around.

Visceral hallucination

Visceral hallucination describes sensations of being pulled or stretched inside the body, often involving specific organs.

Kinaesthetic hallucination
Kinaesthetic hallucinations are false perceptions of joint or muscle sense, e.g. the patient feels his knee vibrating uncontrollably or a calf muscle twisting around his leg.

Olfactory hallucination
Olfactory hallucination is a false perception of smell.

Gustatory hallucination
Gustatory hallucination is a false perception of taste.

Olfactory and gustatory hallucinations frequently occur together because the two senses are difficult to separate.

Other forms of hallucination
Extracampine hallucination
Extracampine hallucination refers to hallucinations experienced outside the normal sensory field of a person, e.g. hearing voices emanating many miles away—often, a delusional explanation for this experience is given.

Functional hallucination
Functional hallucination is where a normal sensory stimulus is required to precipitate a hallucination in that same sensory modality, e.g. the voices are only heard when the doorbell rings.

Reflex hallucination
Reflex hallucination is where a normal sensory stimulus in one modality precipitates a hallucination in another, e.g. the voices are heard when the lights are switched on.

Hypnagogic and hypnopompic hallucinations
Hypnagogic and hypnopompic hallucinations are hallucinations that occur just as a person goes to sleep and awakens, respectively. They may occur normally, but are also commonly seen in sleep disorders (see Chapter 10).

Other perceptual abnormalities
Illusions
Illusions may be defined as misperceptions of external stimuli. They frequently occur in situations of reduced sensory stimulation and consciousness, e.g. a dressing gown is misperceived as a person when one is suddenly awoken in the dark. Alternatively, increased attention and imagination may produce new forms from existing patterns, e.g. the shape of a face may be apparent in a complex fabric pattern— these pareidolic illusions are often secondary to the use of hallucinogenic drugs.

Pseudohallucinations
These may be defined as vivid, involuntary and intrusive images located in inner subjective space, rather than the external sense perceptions of a true hallucination. A good example is the distressing flashbacks that occur in post-traumatic stress disorder (PTSD)—the visions, sounds, or even smells appear real, but are recognized as being generated from within the person's own mind.

Differential diagnosis
A psychosis is characterized by the presence of delusions, hallucinations, or a severe disturbance of behaviour. Typically, the patient's insight into their condition is impaired or absent.

A number of different disorders present with psychotic symptoms. They can often be distinguished by the form and content of either the delusions or hallucinations.

The terms 'psychosis', 'psychotic', 'psychopathic', and 'psychopathy' are used interchangeably by the media, often to sensationalize aggressive or criminal behaviour. Always use the terms precisely: 'psychosis' does not equate to 'dangerousness'. For a definition of 'psychopathy', see Chapter 26.

Psychotic disorders
Schizophrenia

Schizophrenia may be broadly defined as a syndrome characterized by disturbances of thinking, perception, affect, and behaviour, with preserved consciousness and cognitive skills, and not secondary to an identifiable drug or general medical cause.

No single symptom defines schizophrenia; however, the following five have particular diagnostic significance:

- Auditory hallucinations—these can be experienced as thought-echo, hearing thoughts spoken aloud, discussing or giving a running commentary on the patient, or coming from another part of the patient's body (somatic hallucination).
- Delusions of thought-control—thought-insertion, thought-broadcast, thought-withdrawal.
- Delusions of control—passivity of impulse, affect, or volition, or somatic passivity (external influence acting on the body).
- Delusional perception—note that other forms of primary delusion (autochthonous, delusional memory and mood) commonly occur and have diagnostic significance.
- Delusions that are completely impossible—e.g. persecution by knights from the Middle Ages or a belief in the ability to control planetary movements. Note that all other types of delusional content can

occur; often they are secondary to primary delusions or hallucinatory experiences.

Other diagnostic symptoms:

- Other forms of hallucination—note that this includes second-person auditory hallucinations and hallucinations in other sensory modalities; visual hallucinations are rare.
- Thought-disorder (disorder of thought-form)—this is deduced from the way ideas are linked in speech. Several forms are characteristic of schizophrenia (Fig. 5.3). As well as appearing disordered, the thinking process can also appear over-rigid or concrete, e.g. when asked if last month's weight loss has resulted

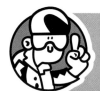

The negative symptoms of schizophrenia can be remembered as the 'five A's':
- Alogia (impaired fluency of speech)
- Affective blunting
- Anhedonia
- Asociality
- Attentional impairment

Forms of thought-disorder characteristic of schizophrenia	
loosening of associations	thoughts appear muddled and lack clarity; in derailment ('Knights move thinking'), unrelated topics of thought jump from one to another, without any linkage – this is quite different to flight of ideas which characterizes mania; in extreme cases, the whole grammatical structure of speech is broken (word salad), or words and phrases are repetitively spoken (verbigeration)
crowding of thought	subjective experience of thoughts concentrated and compressed in the head
thought-blocking	sudden breaks in the train of thought (observed as sudden pauses in speech) which are unaccountable to the patient but may result in the delusional explanation of thought-withdrawal
neologisms	unique words that have particular meaning to the patient, e.g. 'subliminal device'

Fig. 5.3 Forms of thought-disorder characteristic of schizophrenia.

in looser fitting of clothes, the patient angrily retorts that he changes his clothes regularly rather than once a month.

- Catatonic symptoms (see Chapter 13)—these are characterized by excitement, posturing, stupor, negativism, rigidity, waxy flexibility, and command automatism.
- Negative symptoms—this term denotes lack of drive and initiative, social withdrawal, poverty of speech, blunting, and incongruity of affect. These symptoms may be difficult to distinguish from an underlying depressed mood or the effects of psychotropic drugs. Note that delusions and hallucinations in schizophrenia are known as positive symptoms.
- Deterioration in personal behaviour—this may manifest as a lack of personal hygiene, awkward social skills, idleness, impulsivity, or recklessness.

Schizophrenia is diagnosed on the basis of careful identification of either one or more of the first five symptoms (plus any combination of the others); or two or more of the 'other' diagnostic symptoms. The symptoms should be present for at least a month.

Clinical forms of schizophrenia

It is not difficult to imagine the variety of presentations possible with combinations of these symptoms. Various subtypes have been described, based on the predominant pattern of presenting symptoms; however, they are not mutually exclusive. Examples include:

- Paranoid schizophrenia—the clinical picture is dominated by delusions and hallucinations (positive symptoms), with minimal thought-disorder, affective blunting, and negative symptoms.
- Hebephrenic schizophrenia—charcterized by prominent thought-disorder, inappropriate affect, transient delusions and hallucinations, and disturbed behaviour.
- Catatonic schizophrenia—a rare form characterized by predominant catatonic symptoms.
- Residual schizophrenia—predominantly chronic negative symptoms, often following a period of more 'florid' positive symptoms.

Prodromal phase

Before the onset of schizophrenia, many patients show non-specific symptoms and changes in personal functioning such as mild anxiety or depression, abnormalities of speech, eccentric behaviour, and increased social isolation. These changes, usually seen retrospectively, may last for several months.

Delusional disorder

Delusional disorder is closely related to schizophrenia. It is characterized by a single or set of closely related delusions in the absence of any other significant psychopathology or any identifiable physical cause (e.g. alcohol misuse).

Diagnostic guidelines are as follows:

- Delusions are of variable content—commonly, persecution, grandeur, hypochondria, and jealousy.
- Delusions of control and thought-control are excluded (if present, schizophrenia is usually indicated).
- Brief depressive symptoms or hallucinatory experiences may occur.
- The patient has well-preserved personal and social skills, often continuing to lead a normal life.

Traditionally, the following—known as Schneider's First Rank Symptoms—have been used to diagnose schizophrenia:
- **Delusional perception**
- **Delusions of thought-control: withdrawal/insertion/broadcast**
- **Delusions of control: passivity of affect, volition, impulse; influence playing on the body**
- **Auditory hallucinations: third person, running commentary, coming from another part of the body (somatic hallucination) or audible thoughts.**

- Delusions last for at least 3 months and are often long-standing, characteristically developing in mid to late life.

Induced delusional disorder ('folie a deux')

Induced delusional disorder is a rare disorder in which a person with close emotional ties to a person suffering from a delusional disorder (e.g. a sibling) begins to share the delusional ideas themselves. The ideas resolve once the two are separated.

Acute and transient psychotic disorder

Acute and transient psychotic disorder—also known as brief reactive psychosis or schizophreniform psychosis—is commonly precipitated by a life stress, e.g. bereavement. The psychotic symptoms develop rapidly over a period of a few days and do not have a preceding prodromal phase. The symptoms should begin to resolve after one month. When the clinical picture is indistinguishable from schizophrenia, the latter is diagnosed if symptoms perisist for more than one month.

The symptoms should not be secondary to an underlying affective disorder or to a general medical or psychoactive substance cause.

Schizoaffective disorder

In schizoaffective disorder, both definite schizophrenic and definite affective (manic or depressed) symptoms are present simultaneously and occur within several days of each other. It is a controversial category in that it combines the traditionally separate affective and non-affective psychoses. Moreover, it is common for typical symptoms of schizophrenia (e.g. delusions of thought control) to develop in an affective disorder (especially mania), and for affective symptoms (particularly depression) to develop in schizophrenia (post-schizophrenia depression). Therefore it is best to avoid this diagnosis unless an underlying primary affective or schizophrenic disorder cannot be distinguished.

Other differentials

Affective psychoses

Severe depressive episode with psychotic symptoms

Depressive episodes are discussed in Chapter 1.

Delusions encountered in a depressive psychosis are characteristically secondary to, and therefore congruent with, the patient's underlying mood state. Their content commonly involves themes of guilt, unworthiness, illness, infestation, or persecution. Cotard's syndrome is a depressive psychosis characterized by nihilistic delusions, such as a belief that part of the brain has decomposed or that the body no longer exists. As with delusions, hallucinations occur secondarily to depressed mood, and their content is usually congruent with the prevailing mood state. Auditory (usually second-person) and olfactory hallucinations are most common—they may take the form of accusatory or derogatory voices, or the smell of rotting flesh.

Mania with psychotic symptoms (see Chapter 1)

Again, delusions encountered in a manic psychosis are characteristically secondary to the patient's mood state. Delusions of grandeur, persecution, reference, and, occasionally, control occur. The delusions tend to be less fixed and permanent than in the psychotic disorders. The hallucinations (commonly second-person auditory) are usually congruent with the prevailing mood state, e.g. the voices may be telling the person of their great importance. As with depressive disorders, true visual hallucinations are rare, but manic patients often describe a heightened sense of colours or textures—which would be more accurately described as illusions.

Dementia and delirium

Visual hallucinations and paranoid delusions are common in delirium and may occur in dementia, particularly diffuse Lewy body dementia.

Secondary to a general medical condition (organic psychosis) or psychoactive substances

General medical disorders that can cause psychosis are listed in Fig. 5.4. For more information on psychoactive substances, see Chapter 7.

Discussion of vignette

What is Mr DH's diagnosis?

Mr DH presented with a number of bizarre ideas involving themes of persecution (believing he was the victim of government experiments), passivity (believing he was being hypnotized by gamma rays), and

General medical disorders causing psychosis	
System	**Disorder**
neurological	primary/secondary cerebral neoplasms cerebral infarcts epilepsy (especially partial seizures, temporal lobe focus)
endocrinological	hyper/hypothyroidism hyper/hypoparathyroidism hypoadrenocortism (Addison's disease) hypoglycaemia
inflammatory	systemic lupus erythromatosus
metabolic	porphyria
nutritional	B_{12} deficiency
infection	HIV syphilis cerebral abscess
prescribed drugs	anticholinergics antidepressants antiparkinsonian drugs corticosteroids
poisons/toxins	organophosphates fuel/solvents

Fig. 5.4 General medical disorders causing psychosis.

thought-insertion (believing the experiments were introducing images into his mind). The ideas seem fixed and firmly held, and appear to have arisen after he overheard an innocent remark—suggesting delusional perception. In addition, he appears to suffer functional third-person auditory hallucinations reinforcing his beliefs. The combination of these types of delusion and hallucination with apparent deterioration in personal functioning and loss of insight suggest schizophrenia.

The history, mental state, and investigations would need to exclude an underlying mood disorder or psychosis secondary to alcohol or substance abuse. An underlying general medical cause or dementia syndrome, although extremely rare at his age, would need to be excluded by relevant cognitive and physical examinations.

How are delusions elicited?

Delusions may be a presenting symptom when the content of the belief is particularly distressing or significant, e.g. persecution or grandiosity. At other times, their content only becomes apparent through clarification of non-specific complaints such as abnormal behaviour or mood changes, e.g. the patient is restless and anxious because he suddenly believes the world will end. In both situations, there should be detailed enquiry by the examiner and careful monitoring for any cues in the history, such as remarks by the patient that they feel afraid or notice things differently to before.

It is useful to develop a number of opening questions to explore specific delusional themes. For example:
- Persecution—'Does anyone seem to be trying to harm you in anyway, spying on you, or trying to kill or poison you?'
- Reference—'Do people seem to drop hints meant for you or say things with double meanings, or do you hear messages for yourself from the television or radio?'
- Grandeur—'Do you feel you have any special powers or a special mission in life?'
- Delusion of control—'Do you feel that your will has been replaced by that of a power or force outside yourself?'

If the patient appears to be deluded, the following points need to be clarified:
- Is the belief personal or shared?
- What is the evidence for the belief?
- How long has the patient had the belief and how did it begin?
- Could the patient be wrong?

How are hallucinations elicited?

Hallucinations are similar to delusions in that the patient often does not have any insight into the abnormality of their experience—this is particularly true in the acute phase of a psychotic illness. Again, one must look out for cues in the history, such as complaints of persecution (e.g. being followed or monitored) or of others criticizing or talking about them (especially if this occurs when alone or after going to bed). The patient may also appear distracted or preoccupied by something else in their surroundings.

If the patient does describe perceptual experiences suggesting a hallucination, or simply complains of 'hearing voices', the following should be clarified:

37

- What exactly is the content of their experience?
- What initiates or stops the experience? Is it involuntary?
- Is the experience perceived in external space?
- Is the experience personal or shared?
- Does the patient feel they could be misinterpreting other stimuli or imagining their experience? If not, do they believe a special mechanism explains their experience?

To maintain rapport with the patient and lessen any suspicions they may have, direct questioning about perceptual disturbances requires a sensitive and non-prejudicial approach—for example: 'We ask this question of everyone, and would like to ask you . . . Do you ever hear noises or voices when there is nobody about and no ordinary explanation seems possible? . . . Do you see or feel things other people cannot?'.

6. Memory Loss and Confusion

Mrs ML, a 68-year-old patient on a medical ward, was referred for a psychiatric assessment. The medical staff had observed considerable restlessness and confusion since her admission for pneumonia. Although her physical illness had been successfully treated, she continued to get lost on the ward and believed she was staying at home with her sister who had died several years previously. When her relatives were interviewed, they described a recent deterioration in her memory; by this they meant difficulty remembering the date, getting lost on her way to the shops, and forgetting to turn the oven off. She had become more irritable in mood, accusing her family of stealing her money, and had mistaken her grandchildren for her own brothers and sisters.

Psychopathology

Disturbances of cognition (attention, orientation, memory, judgement) and their underlying causes form the basis of this chapter.

Memory impairment

Memory is stored in three ways:
- Immediate.
- Short term.
- Long term.

Both immediate and short-term memory are influenced by the level of attention the observer pays to external stimuli.

Immediate (sensory store)

In the immediate store, visual and auditory information is held for less than a second in the form it is perceived.

Short term (primary or working memory)

Information in the short-term store is held for up to 30 seconds and usually comprises a maximum of six or seven items which are held for current use.

Long term (secondary memory)

All memory stored beyond the short term store is classified as long term memory; this can range from a minute to many years. It is abnormalities of this form of memory that make up the various amnesic or dysmnesic syndromes. Two mechanisms of storage are described:
- Semantic memory—this includes vocabulary, facts, and concepts without specification in time and place, e.g. the Queen's name.
- Episodic memory—this includes personally experienced events, e.g. recent incidents in hospital.

This form of memory is also categorized in terms of :
- Ability to learn new material or anterograde memory—often (confusingly) termed short-term memory.
- Recent memory—e.g. news events 1 week ago.
- Remote memory—e.g. news events 10 years ago.

- Retrograde amnesia—loss of episodic memory that was formed prior to a brain insult, e.g. head injury; this differs from post-traumatic amnesia which refers to loss of memory for events after the brain insult.

Memory impairment is usually associated with the amnesic and dementia syndromes.

Amnesic syndrome
The amnesic syndrome is an acquired disorder of memory and is characterized by:
- Marked impairment in the ability to learn new material.
- Loss of memory for recent and remote events in reverse order of their occurrence.
- No impairment of consciousness or other intellectual functions.

This disorder is usually secondary to lesions in the limbic (especially hippocampal) or diencephalic regions of the brain (Fig 6.1).

Because of the memory loss, patients are frequently disorientated in time and place (although rarely in person) and have no insight into their problems. The following symptoms may also occur:
- Confabulation—falsification of memory in the context of clear consciousness and caused by an organic impairment of memory. It is distinct from delusional memory and delusional retrospective falsification of memory, which occur in psychotic disorders.
- Perseveration—a verbal or motor response appropriate to the first question or instruction but inappropriate to those that follow: for example, when asked the year, the patient says '1998'; when later asked the Queen's name, '1998' is repeated.

It must be stressed that other areas of intellectual function such as reading and comprehension skills are intact. It is not unusual for these patients to present as entirely normal, with a confabulated recent history only emerging after careful examination of memory in the mental state.

Dementia syndrome
The dementia syndrome is an acquired global impairment of intellect, memory, and personality, without impairment of consciousness, and is usually chronic and progressive in its course.

This disorder is usually secondary to a variety of diffuse brain pathologies, but is occasionally secondary to treatable general medical causes.

Main categories of impairment
Dementia is a global impairment of function rather than a specific loss of memory. The main categories of impairment are:

Memory impairment This follows the pattern of the amnesic syndrome, with impairment of new learning and recent memory most prominent, leading to disorientation.

Language impairment Both expressive and receptive dysphasias may occur, manifested by difficulties comprehending commands or by vague speech; ultimately, the patient may become mute.

Apraxia Difficulties executing complex motor activities (such as putting a letter in an envelope).

Agnosia Failure to recognize familiar objects or people despite intact sensory function.

Abnormalities of higher intellectual function e.g. difficulties with planning and sequencing complex activities, judgement, and abstract thinking.

Changes in personality and behaviour e.g. loss of drive, increased apathy, and social withdrawal. At the other extreme, the patient may become more socially disinhibited, hostile, or aggressive. Changes in mood may also occur, such as depression or euphoria.

Psychotic symptoms Visual hallucinations are particularly common and they are often accompanied by persecutory delusions.

Deterioration in personal functioning Personal relationships, social functioning, activities of daily living (such as personal hygiene, food preparation), and occupational functioning decline.

Loss of motor and sensory functioning This is usually seen in the later stages of a dementia and leads, for instance, to blindness, paralysis, and urinary incontinence.

As with the amnesic syndrome, insight into the illness is lost, except in the early stages. Evidence of symptoms should be present for at least 6 months before a diagnosis is made.

The pattern of functional deficit can indicate which part of the brain is primarily affected by the pathology (Fig. 6.2).

Primary neurodegenerative causes of dementia

Alzheimer's disease The gross pathology of Alzheimer's disease is characterized by generalized atrophy of the brain, with widened sulci and ventricles; the frontal and temporal lobes are particularly affected.

Features of cellular pathology comprise:

Causes of amnesic syndrome	
Diencephalic damage	third ventricle tumours/cysts bilateral thalamic infarction post subarachnoid haemorrhage vitamin B_1 deficiency (Korsakov's syndrome): • chronic alcohol abuse (see Chapter 7) • gastric carcinoma • severe malnutrition • hyperemesis gravidarum
Hippocampal damage	carbon monoxide poisoning (anoxia) herpes simplex virus encephalitis closed head injury bilateral posterior cerebral artery occlusion

Fig. 6.1 Causes of amnesic syndrome.

Focal lobe deficits	
Lobe	**Deficit**
frontal	expressive dysphasia contralateral spastic paresis reduced fine motor control difficulties initiating and planning activities apathy, slowing of thought (dorsolateral pre-frontal cortical lesions) disinhibition, facetious humour (orbito-frontal lesions) primitive reflexes
temporal	receptive dysphasia memory disturbance cortical deafness visuospatial difficulties, e.g. inability to recognise faces (prosopagnosia) personality change and psychosis
parietal	receptive dysphasia apraxia/agnosia sensory inattention/neglect right/left disorientation agraphia (inability to write), dyscalculia (inability to perform mathematical tasks)
occipital	cortical blindness loss of visual perception

Fig. 6.2 Focal lobe deficits.

- Extracellular senile plaques in cortical and subcortical grey matter—these consist of a core of β-amyloid surrounded by filamentous material.
- Intracellular neurofibrillary tangles resulting from abnormal phosphorylation of tau protein.
- Intracellular cytoplasmic vacuoles (granulovacuolar degeneration) in the hippocampus.
- Amyloid deposition in the blood vessel walls.

Clinically, Alzheimer's disease characteristically has an insidious onset and a slowly progressive course. Early symptoms include impairment of new learning, loss of recent memory, and resultant disorientation in time and place. Personality and behaviour changes may also occur at this stage. Aphasia, apraxia, agnosia, and motor abnormalities develop later.

Vascular dementia (multi-infarct dementia) The brain may appear normal in size or atrophied with ventricular dilatation. Dementia may arise from a single cerebral infarct, although in most cases the infarcts are multiple. The usual cause is cerebral atherosclerosis and the white matter of the brain is particularly vulnerable to ischaemia.

The characteristic clinical picture is of abrupt onset and stepwise deterioration. The course and pattern of cognitive deficits are highly variable and depend on the location of the infarcts. Patients with vascular dementia are more likely to demonstrate focal neurological signs (e.g. exaggerated tendon reflexes) and preserve their underlying personality than are patients with Alzheimer's disease.

Pick's disease In Pick's disease, atrophy is concentrated on the frontal and temporal lobes—so-called knife-blade atrophy (due to the appearance of atrophied gyri). Microscopically, there is neuronal loss and astrocytic proliferation. In addition, swollen balloon cells and intracellular Pick's bodies occur.

Clinically, there is prominent early development of frontal lobe signs such as behavioural disinhibition, deteriorating social skills, apathy, and language abnormalities. Memory loss and apraxias occur at a later stage.

Huntington's disease This is associated with atrophy of the frontal lobe, parietal lobe, basal ganglia (caudate and putamen), and ventricular dilatation.

Clinically, Huntington's disease has an insidious onset, initially presenting with non-specific motor signs (e.g. twitching, grimacing, clumsiness) or subtle changes in personality or mood (e.g. anxiety, irritability, suspiciousness, social neglect). Depressed mood is common; occasionally patients may present with a depressive psychosis. Memory problems, impaired judgement, and slowed speed of thought may occur early; severe memory loss, disorientation, and loss of insight tend to develop later. The movement disorder develops into a severe syndrome of extrapyramidal (chorea, tics, ballismus), pyramidal (weakness and spasticity), and cerebellar (ataxia, wide-based gait, intention tremor) abnormalities.

Creutzfeldt–Jakob disease (CJD) Abnormalities in CJD result from the transmissible prion (proteinaceous particle) which gives rise to a subacute spongiform encephalopathy. This is characterized by neuronal loss, astrocytic proliferation and vacuolation of cell bodies, the latter giving rise to a 'spongiform' appearance.

Clinically, there is often a vague prodromal illness characterized by fatigue, apathy, anxiety, concentration problems, or sleep problems. This is rapidly followed by profound cognitive deterioration and a syndrome of severe extrapyramidal, pyramidal, and cerebellar abnormalities. Myoclonus is particularly common.

Parkinson's disease/diffuse Lewy body disease In Parkinson's disease there is significant loss of pigmented dopaminergic neurons in the substantia nigra region of the basal ganglia and loss of cholinergic neurons. The neuronal loss appears to be secondary to intracellular eosinophilic structures called Lewy Bodies.

In addition to the classic extrapyramidal movement disorder, a progressive dementia syndrome occurs in approximately 20–60% of patients and this may be complicated by coexistent depressive symptoms.

Recently, a form of dementia has been described that is secondary to diffuse cortical and subcortical Lewy bodies. This is characterized by:
- Progressive but often-fluctuating cognitive impairment.
- Frequent falls.
- Changes in consciousness.
- Vivid visual hallucinations and paranoid delusions.

Extrapyramidal symptoms may not occur until late in the course of the disease.

HIV dementia Direct involvement of the brain occurs in about 50% of AIDS cases and is characterized by diffuse multifocal destruction of subcortical structures and white matter. The dementia syndrome is characterized by apathy, poor concentration, slowness of thought, memory loss, and, occasionally, psychotic symptoms. In addition, weakness of limbs occurs, leading to a paraparesis, tremor, ataxia, and double incontinence.

Subcortical causes of dementia

A clinical picture of dementia has been described when the neuronal degeneration primarily affects subcortical structures, e.g. basal ganglia. Typically, there is slowing of cognition due to imparied attention and vigilance. Apparent memory difficulties often respond to observer prompting. Other features include mood disturbance, psychosis, and difficulty with complex intellectual tasks. This presentation may closely resemble non-organic psychiatric disorders, e.g. depression with psychomotor retardation.

Diseases likely to cause this presentation include: Parkinson's disease, Huntington's disease, Progressive supranuclear palsy, Vascular dementia, HIV, and Wilson's diease.

General medical disorders and drugs causing dementia

The general medical disorders and drugs that can cause dementia are listed in Fig. 6.3.

Causes of dementia: general medical disorders and drugs	
System	**Cause**
neurological/degenerative	subdural haematoma diffuse and/or focal brain injury intracranial tumour hydrocephalus progressive supranuclear palsy multiple sclerosis head injury
metabolic	Wilson's disease chronic uraemia and dialysis chronic hepatic encephalopathy
infection	neurosyphilis trypanosomiasis
anoxia	carbon monoxide poisoning
endocrine	hypothyroidism hypoparathyroidism
nutritional	pellagra (Niacin deficiency) subacute combined degeneration of the cord (B_{12} deficiency)
inflammatory	systemic lupus erythematosus polyarteritis nodosa
poisons	mercury manganese
drugs/substance abuse	alcohol solvents barbiturates and benzodiazepines

Fig. 6.3 Causes of dementia: general medical disorders and drugs.

Confusion

Consciousness refers to the state of awareness of the self and the environment.

Three areas of functioning are closely related to the level of consciousness:

- Attention—the focusing of consciousness on a particular person, object, or event.
- Concentration—the maintenance of attention on a particular person, object, or event.
- Orientation—an awareness of time, place, and self in their current situation (it is affected by impaired consciousness and memory).

Disturbances of consciousness

A disturbance of consciousness implies an underlying

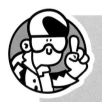

Confusion refers to an inability to think clearly and coherently. It usually pertains to the acute disturbances in consciousness and cognition which form the basis of this section, but could also apply to the presentation of psychosis or severe anxiety encountered previously. As it is so non-specific, it is a term best avoided.

organic disorder, or the involvement of a psychoactive substance.

Clear consciousness

This is the level of normal consciousness. States of heightened consciousness may occur, in which there is a subjective sense of greater awareness (e.g. colours appear more vivid). These usually occur at times of heightened emotions, such as falling in love or during hypomania, and can also occur with stimulant or hallucinogenic drugs. The dementia syndrome occurs in the presence of clear consciousness.

Clouding of consciousness

Clouding of consciousness is the mildest form of impairment, with subtle changes in attention, concentration, orientation, comprehension, judgement, and memory. The patient may appear drowsy or, at the other extreme, agitated. This state is easily overlooked and may require prolonged observation.

Drowsiness

At the stage of drowsiness, the patient's speech is slurred and they will drift into unconsciousness without sensory stimulation. Reflexes and muscle tone are reduced.

Sopor

At the stage of sopor, the patient is unconscious and can be aroused only by strong stimulation. (It is not the same as stupor—see Chapter 13.)

Coma

Coma is the most extreme disturbance of consciousness: the patient is unconscious and unrousable; reflexes and muscle tone are greatly reduced and breathing is slowed down.

Delirium

Delirium is a syndrome characterized by fluctuating disturbances of consciousness accompanied by changes in perception, thinking, memory, affect, psychomotor activity, and the sleep–wake cycle.

It is also known (rather confusingly!) as acute confusional state, acute organic reaction, and toxic confusional state.

There are a number of causes (Fig. 6.4). The syndrome usually begins within hours or days, but sometimes (e.g. in the case of head injury) begins abruptly. The course is usually short, resolving as the underlying cause resolves. In exceptional cases (such as bacterial endocarditis and chronic liver disease) it may last much longer.

Evidence of the following abnormalities are required to make the diagnosis.

Impaired consciousness

This most commonly manifests as clouding of consciousness, with resultant impairment in attention and concentration—the patient is easily distracted and may display perseveration (failure to shift attention).

Global disturbance of cognition

This involves impairment of short-term memory, disorientation, impaired judgement, and impaired abstract thinking. Perceptual disturbances are common, ranging from simple misinterpretations (e.g. a door slamming is mistaken for an explosion), to illusions (e.g. a crack in the wall is perceived as a snake), to true hallucinations. The latter are usually visual in their sensory modality—a form rarely encountered in the psychotic disorders. Transient delusions, usually persecutory, often derive from these visual images.

Psychomotor disturbances

A variety of fluctuating hypoactive and hyperactive states may occur; speech may become pressured, incoherent, or rambling, and the patient may show an enhanced startle reaction.

Disturbance of the sleep–wake cycle

This can range from insomnia, daytime drowsiness, and night-time hyperactivity, to complete reversal of the normal cycle. Disturbing dreams may occur and symptoms in general are worse at night (lucid intervals during the day are common).

Disturbances of affect

Again, this varies enormously; depression, elation, suspiciousness, anxiety, fear, and perplexity may occur.

Differential diagnosis
Dementia or delirium?

Delirium frequently complicates a dementia, and the two may coexist. For example, a patient with early Alzheimer's disease is admitted to a medical ward because of a urinary tract infection which precipitates a delirium; the underlying cognitive deficit can be assessed only once the delirium has resolved.

Dementia syndromes such as the vascular and the diffuse Lewy body type can resemble a delirium at times because of their more fluctuant course; this is particularly true of the latter owing to the common visual hallucinations and nocturnal worsening in cognitive functioning. See Fig. 6.5.

Dementia and delirium secondary to the effects of alcohol and substance misuse

These are described in Chapter 7.

Fig. 6.4 Causes of delirium. MAOI= monoamine oxidase inhibitor.

System	Cause
Causes of delirium	
neurological/degenerative	subdural haematoma intracranial tumour head injury* subarachnoid haemorrhage cerebral infarct/ischaemia epilepsy*
infection	cerebral abscess meningitis encephalitis* bronchopneumonia urinary tract infection septicaemia endocarditis tropical infections, e.g. malaria
endocrine	hypo/hyperthyroidism* hypo/hyperparathyroidism hypo/hyperadrenocorticism (Cushing's, Addison's disease)* hypoglycaemia* hypopituatarism
prescribed drugs	digoxin steroids* anticonvulsants benzodiazepines tricyclic and MAOI antidepressants anticholinergics L-dopa salicylates isoniazid
metabolic	electrolyte disturbance uraemia hepatic encephalopathy porphyria
nutritional	pellagra (Niacin deficiency) B_{12} deficiency B_1 (thiamine) deficiency
poisons	lead mercury manganese
anoxia	heart failure respiratory failure

(*indicates those conditions described in greater detail in the text)

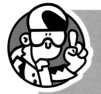

It is important to differentiate the common syndromes of dementia and delirium because of their different causes and prognoses. Learn Fig. 6.5 well.

Psychotic disorders

The disturbed behaviour, distractibility, and thought-disorder of acute psychoses may resemble delirium. The negative symptoms of schizophrenia may resemble the cognitive dysfunction of dementia. However, when the patient is co-operative, careful assessment of cognitive functioning is normal in both situations.

Depressive disorder

Pseudodementia is the term given when a patient with a severe depressive disorder appears to have significant cognitive problems. It is due to the effects of psychomotor retardation, poor concentration, and ideas of worthlessness (Fig. 6.6). Unlike dementia, the apparent cognitive dysfunction improves with treatment of the depression.

Dissociative states

Dissociative states, particularly dissociative amnesia and fugue, present with apparent cognitive abnormalities similar to dementia or delirium. However, they usually develop suddenly after a psychological stress and the dysfunction is atypical for organic disorders, e.g. the patient 'loses their identity' whereas other cognitive functions are intact (see Fig. 6.6).

Hypomania and mania

The disturbed behaviour and distractibility of hypomania and mania can give the impression of a delirium; however, cognitive assessment is normal when the patient co-operates.

Factors differentiating delirium from dementia		
Feature	Delirium	Dementia
onset	acute	insidious
duration	hours–weeks	months–years
course	fluctuating	progressive
consciousness	impaired	normal
orientation	impaired	impaired

memory:
1. short term (<30 s)
2. long term:
    new learning
    recent/remote
	impaired
	
	impaired
	usually intact
		usually normal
		
		impaired
		impaired in latter stages

perceptual disturbances	common	occur in latter stages
sleep–wake cycle	disrupted	usually normal

Fig. 6.5 Factors differentiating delirium from dementia.

Memory loss associated with dementia, pseudodementia of depressive disorders, and dissociative states		
Dementia	Pseudodementia	Dissociative amnesia
preceding cognitive deterioration	preceding/prevailing depressed mood	sudden loss of memory following acute stress
cognitive abnormalities demonstrated	patient often unwilling to answer questions	memory loss specific and atypical
usually little insight into cognitive problems	patient often complains of memory loss or state they cannot answer the questions	classically demonstrate 'belle indifference' to their dysfunction
attention/concentration may be impaired	attention and concentrationmay be impaired	attention/concentration intact

Fig. 6.6 Memory loss associated with dementia, pseudodementia of depressive disorders, and dissociative states.

Generalized anxiety disorder

In patients with generalized anxiety disorder, resultant poor attention and concentration during the interview and mental state examination may give the impression of cognitive problems.

Learning disability

These disorders are described in Chapter 11.

Organic mental and personality disorders

This is a large collection of disorders which along with dementia, delirium, and amnesic syndromes, complete the various 'organic disorders' encountered in psychiatry. They are similar in presentation to the other psychiatric (or functional) disorders described in Part I, The Patient Presents With. However, in each case the disorder is directly caused by a recognised physical disease or injury. The important forms are:

- Organic mood disorder (see Chapter 1).
- Organic anxiety disorder (see Chapter 2).
- Organic hallucinosis (see Chapter 5).
- Organic delusional (schizophrenia-like) disorder (see Chapter 5).
- Organic catatonic disorder (see Chapter 13).
- Organic personality disorder (see Chapter 8).

In common with the functional disorders they resemble, they differ from delirium and dementia in that there is preservation of consciousness and other cognitive functions.

General medical conditions of special significance to psychiatry

There are many physical diseases or injuries which can cause psychiatric symptoms: the following section describes those which have particular relevance to psychiatry and often feature in the differential diagnoses.

Complex partial seizures, temporal lobe focus

Complex partial seizures with a temporal lobe focus—popularly known as temporal lobe epilepsy (TLE)—can give rise to many psychiatric symptoms. As with generalized (tonic-clonic or grand mal) seizures, there is impairment of consciousness and five stages occur:

- Prodrome (hours to days)—increased irritability, low mood, and apprehension are some of the non-specific changes reported, along with physical feelings of flushing, pallor, and dyspepsia.
- Aura (seconds to minutes)—where there is a temporal lobe focus, a complex range of symptoms occur, including hallucinations in any modality, depersonalization and derealization, any affective symptom, and disturbances of thought such as crowding of thought, thought blocking, and intrusive thoughts. In addition, common physical complaints include lip smacking, stomach churning, and flushing or pallor.
- Seizure (minutes)—during this period there is impaired consciousness and a psychomotor disturbance usually characterized by stereotypical, repetitive behaviour such as grimacing; or more complex goal-directed behaviour known as automatisms (such as driving a car). Rarely, more prolonged twilight states occur, lasting up to a few weeks, during which delusions and hallucinations may be evident. Secondary generalization to a tonic-clonic seizure may occur.
- Post-ictal (hours)—during recovery, disorientation, memory loss, agitation, and irritability occur.
- Inter-ictal—a prolonged psychosis may develop.

Head injury

The psychiatric disturbances associated with head injury can be divided into three time-frames:

- Immediate—impairment of consciousness, delirium, and retrograde or anterograde amnesia.
- Short term—Post-Concussional Syndrome, characterized by sleep problems, fatigue, poor concentration, memory problems, depression, anxiety, a low tolerance to stress, and an increased risk of alcohol misuse. There are physical complaints of headache and dizziness.
- Long term—a chronic cognitive deficit is more likely if there is a long period of post-traumatic amnesia; repeated head injury through boxing can give rise to a progressive dementia (dementia pugilistica) with a similar pathology to Alzheimer's disease. Another long-term sequela is organic personality disorder, particularly with frontal lobe damage, giving rise to a syndrome of greater impulsivity (inability to persevere with tasks), emotional lability, increased aggressive behaviour, inappropriate social and sexual behaviour, and language difficulties. Finally, there is

an increased likelihood of affective and non-affective psychosis, particularly depressive psychosis. Note that the suicide rate rises to 14 times the normal rate.

Encephalitis
Although largely presenting with characteristic neurological symptoms, encephalitis may rarely present as a typical functional psychiatric illness before progressing to impairment of consciousness and delirium. Chronically, it may give rise to an organic personality disorder or a postencephalitic syndrome characterized by apathy or irritability, cognitive difficulties, and sleep and eating problems.

HIV
In addition to the dementia syndrome described in the previous chapter, the direct neuropathology of HIV—with or without the effect of opportunistic neurological infections and neoplasms—can give rise to a delirium, an organic affective, or organic psychotic disorder.

Syphilis
Similarly to HIV, tertiary syphilis ('general paralysis of the insane') may present with a dementia, delirium, organic affective, or organic psychotic disorder.

Thyroid disease
Hyperthyroidism characteristically presents with anxiety, irritability, and overactivity. It occasionally causes a delirium ('thyroid storm'), but is only rarely associated with mania or a non-affective psychosis. Hypothyroidism characteristically causes apathy and fatigue; it may cause an organic affective (depressive) disorder or give rise to a dementia.

Glucocorticoid disease
Cushing's syndrome frequently gives rise to an organic affective disorder (depression more than mania), but can (rarely) cause delirium, dementia, or an organic psychosis. In contrast, steroid treatment usually causes elation rather than depressed mood. Addison's disease can also cause organic mood, anxiety, and psychotic disorders in addition to dementia and delirium (particularly as a feature of acute adrenal crisis).

Hypoglycaemia
Subacute and chronic forms of hypoglycaemia (e.g. as a result of insulinoma) can give rise to apathy, social withdrawal, organic personality change, and periods of delirium and dementia.

Discussion of vignette
Mrs ML's diagnosis?
The long-term history of Mrs ML suggested a number of cognitive abnormalities, namely poor new and recent memory (forgetting to turn her oven off, not knowing the date, losing things around the house), topographical agnosia (losing her way on familiar routes), and visual agnosia (misidentifying her grandchildren). Accusing her family of stealing money may have represented increased suspiciousness or delusional ideas of persecution. More marked behaviour disturbance occurred when she was admitted to hospital with a physical illness. It seems likely that the chronic cognitive dysfunction of a dementia syndrome was exacerbated by a comorbid delirium caused by her chest infection. Even without a delirium, sudden changes of environment cause more pronounced disorientation in dementia.

Assessment of cognitive dysfunction
What factors in the history are important?
An accurate corroborative history, from relatives, friends, or ward staff, is vital to establish the course and pattern of symptoms. Consider:
- Is there fluctuation and periods of lucidity?
- What and when were the first observed problems?
- How did the problems progress—insidiously, stepwise, reaching stability?
- What effect do the problems have on the patient's family, and social and occupational life?

Develop a checklist of situations and other activities of daily living to assess their impairment. An easy-to-remember daily timetable can be used (i.e. dressing, washing, using the toilet, running a bath, cleaning the house, ability to go to the shops, handling money, preparing hot meals, social and recreational activities, ability to drive, and performance at work).
Finally, always try to establish:
- The level of premorbid functioning, e.g. difficulty managing finances may be a more significant symptom for an accountant compared to a person always dependent on their spouse.
- An accurate medical and drug history.
- The presence of any new physical symptoms, particularly if they appear neurological in origin.

How is cognitive dysfunction assessed on mental state examination?

The following should be asked in all mental state examinations.

Orientation

Ask the patient:
- Day, date, month, year, time of day.
- Current location (e.g. ward number, floor of building), town, country.
- Their own name and age, and the identity of a familiar person (e.g. doctor, nurse).

Attention and concentration

Ask the patient to do one of the following:
- Repeat the months of the year backwards.
- Subtract 7 from 100 and then keep subtracting 7 from the number they are left with (serial 7s) until they reach fewer than 10.

Note the time it takes to complete the task and any mistakes made.

Remember that the serial 7s is also a test of arithmetical ability: if necessary, adjust to the expected intellect of the patient (i.e. if too easy, try serial 13s from 500; if too hard, try serial 3s from 20).

Primary memory

Ask the patient to repeat a sequence of digits building up from 3 to 6 numbers immediately after they have been told (digit span test): e.g. 3-6-1, 5-9-4-8, 6-7-4-1-3, 9-2-3-5-8-6. Normal = ±6.

Secondary memory

Learn new information (short term memory). Ask the patient to repeat the name and address of a fictitious person 5 minutes after they have been told: e.g. John Brown, 8 Market St, Sheffield 7.

Ensure they have registered the information by asking them to repeat the address immediately after they have been told, but do not warn them they will be tested later (to prevent rehearsal). Record the number of address items recalled.

Recent memory Ask the patient to recall recent (in the last few days) news or sporting events, or other recent events you can independently verify.

Remote memory Ask the patient facts such as the names of the present and previous Prime Ministers, or personal details such as previous addresses if they can be independently verified.

Cognitive assessment of delirium typically demonstrates impairment of orientation, the digit span test, concentration tests, and memory for new information. In dementia, impairment of orientation, memory for new information, and recent memory is typical.

Intelligence

Finally it is important to make a subjective assessment of the patient's intelligence based on their history (e.g. educational achievements) and performance in the interview (e.g. vocabulary, general knowledge). A simple bedside test is to ask the patient to name as many parts of face as possible.

Additional tests of cognitive functioning
Frontal lobe function

Assessment of frontal lobe function comprises:
- Verbal fluency—ask the patient to give as many words as they can starting with a certain letter (e.g. F, T) or belonging to a certain category (e.g. four-legged animals) in 1 minute. They should achieve more than 20 to exclude significant frontal lobe dysfunction; exclude any words repeated.
- Abstract thinking—ask the patient to estimate measurements such as the length of a train or the height of the Eiffel Tower; ask them to interpret similarities, e.g. between an orange and a pear, or a car and a bicycle.
- Motor sequencing—ask the patient to repeat a sequenced hand movement, e.g. a fist, slapping and slicing movement to the words 'punch, slop, cut', allowing the patient to continue after stopping (in frontal lobe lesions these are often poorly co-ordinated).

Parietal lobe function

Assessment of parietal lobe function comprises:

- Complex movement (praxis)—ask the patient to take a piece of paper in their left hand, fold it in half, and place it on their right knee.
- Check right-left orientation; ask to complete a mathematical sum (acalculia) and ask to write a sentence (agraphia).
- Constructional abilities—ask the patient to copy a prepared drawing, usually overlapping pentagons, or ask them to draw a clock face stating a time for the hands (this also tests for extrapersonal neglect).
- Object recognition (asteriognosis)—ask the patient to name a coin placed blindly in their palm.

Language (mixture of frontal and parietal lobe functions)

Ask the patient to:

- Name nearby objects.
- Repeat a prepared sentence.

A thorough physical examination and relevant physical investigations complete the assessment process and are particularly important whenever an organic cause is suspected (see Chapter 14).

A useful screening tool for dementia is the Mini-Mental State Examination (MMSE; Fig. 6.7). This standardized set of questions can be incorporated to screen for or monitor the progress of a dementia. A score below 25/30 suggests dementia; 25–27/30 is borderline.

Mini-Mental State Examination	
1) year, season, date, day, month, county, town, country, place, floor level	10
2) immediate recall of words, e.g. apple, table, penny	3
3) serial 7s, stop after five answers	5
4) name two objects, e.g. pencil, watch	2
5) repeat: 'No ifs, ands or buts'	1
6) follow the three-step paper folding command	3
7) read aloud and obey the written statement 'close your eyes'	1
8) write a sentence	1
9) copy prepared design (overlapping pentagons)	1
10) ask patient to repeat words from 2) (ensure 5 min elapsed)	3
	30

Fig. 6.7 Mini-Mental State Examination.

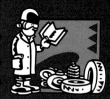

7. Alcohol and Drugs

ALCOHOL AND SUBSTANCE MISUSE

Ms AD, aged 45, is referred to the psychiatric outpatient clinic for advice on treating excessive alcohol consumption. She had presented to her GP with complaints of 'depression and anxiety', but during the interview it had emerged that she regularly drank six cans of strong lager plus half a bottle of wine per day. She had gradually increased her consumption after her divorce, and had been drinking on a daily basis since she lost her job 2 years ago. She usually drank alone, in her house, beginning as soon as she got up in the morning. When she did not drink, she became anxious and irritable, developed a hand tremor, and had a strong desire to obtain alcohol. Matters had culminated recently when she had had a seizure after recovering from routine surgery. Her previous attempt to stop drinking, 6 months ago, had led to a 2-week period of abstinence.

Psychopathology
Alcohol
Alcohol is a widely used recreational drug because of its relaxing and disinhibiting effects. It is also an extremely common cause of physical and psychiatric morbidity. The psychiatric manifestations of alcohol use will form the basis of this chapter, providing the conceptual framework of all substance-related disorders.

Mechanism of action
The biochemical action of alcohol is complex and only partly understood. It has a number of effects on the various neurotransmitter systems of the brain. The primary effects are thought to be stimulation of inhibitory gamma-aminobutyric acid (GABA) receptors and inhibition of excitatory glutamate receptors, causing sedation, relief of anxiety, and amnesia. In addition, alcohol appears to affect noradrenergic, dopaminergic, serotoninergic and opioid systems, giving rise to other effects such as nausea, euphoria, and craving.

Metabolism
Approximately 75% of metabolism takes place in the liver. There are two mechanisms:
- Alcohol dehydrogenase converts alcohol to acetaldehyde; this is then converted to acetate by acetaldehyde dehydrogenase.
- Mixed-function oxidases metabolize alcohol within the endoplasmic reticulum of hepatocytes.

Clinical syndromes caused by excessive use of alcohol and other psychoactive substances
Acute intoxication
Acute intoxication is the most common manifestation of alcohol use and will be suffered by most medical students at some point. The term denotes the acute dose-related effects of a substance which resolve once the substance (or its active metabolites) are expelled from the body.

In the case of alcohol, which is a CNS depressant, low blood alcohol concentrations produce an enhanced sense of wellbeing, greater confidence, relief of anxiety, and social disinhibition. Mood changes vary and include depression, elation, and aggression. Visual reaction times are reduced and motor coordination becomes impaired. As blood alcohol levels increase, coordination, judgement, and level of consciousness deteriorate, leading to ataxia, disorientation, amnesia, incontinence, and eventually death secondary to respiratory depression.

Pathological intoxication

The term 'pathological intoxication' denotes the rare syndrome of uncharacteristic violent or aggressive behaviour after drinking small quantities of alcohol that would not cause intoxication in most people.

Harmful use

The term 'harmful use' describes the secondary damaging effects of alcohol or other psychoactive substance misuse.

Using alcohol to illustrate, a number of consequences may result:

- Physical—alcohol adversely affects most systems of the body (Fig. 7.1).
- Psychological—increased alcohol consumption gives rise to a range of symptoms and behaviours, such as increased depressive symptoms and violence. These are discussed in more detail in the discussion of differential diagnosis.

Medical complications of excessive alcohol use	
System	**Complication**
neurological	epilepsy—alcohol withdrawal head injury cerebellar degeneration polyneuropathy delirium tremens/Wernicke's encephalopathy/Korsakoff's syndrome*
cardiovascular	hypertension cardiomyopathy arrthymias ischaemic heart disease
gastrointestinal	acute gastritis carcinoma oesophagus/rectum pancreatitis haemochromatosis alcoholic hepatitis/cirrhosis
metabolic	hyperuricaemia hyperlipidaemia hypoglycaemia hypomagnesaemia
respiratory	pneumonia
endocrine	pseudo-Cushing's syndrome
musculoskeletal	acute and chronic myopathy osteoporosis osteomalacia
haemopoeitic	macrocytosis thrombocytopaenia leukopaenia
reproduction	small babies foetal alcohol syndrome: • small stature • low birth weight • intellectual impairment • facial abnormality • overactivity

Fig. 7.1 Medical complications of excessive alcohol use (*more detail in text).

- Social—this might include increased absenteeism from work, increased financial difficulties or debt, recurrent drink-driving offences, and problems sustaining relationships.

Dependence syndrome

Whereas the previous disorder may occur with sporadic rather than regular consumption, a dependence syndrome develops against a backdrop of heavy, regular consumption. Diagnosis depends on identification of three or more of the following:

- Compulsion to take the substance—this involves an intense desire or craving to take the substance after the original effects have ceased.
- Stereotyped pattern of substance use—e.g. the dependent drinker drinks at particular times of day owing to difficulties exerting control over intake (because of withdrawal symptoms).
- Physiological withdrawal symptoms—with alcohol (a CNS depressant) the withdrawal symptoms are those of CNS excitation: tremor ('the shakes'), restlessness, agitation, sweating, nausea, anxiety, tachycardia, pyrexia, hypertension, pupil dilatation, and insomnia. Occasionally, seizures occur. Withdrawal symptoms frequently begin after waking from sleep (as the previous night's blood alcohol concentration has decreased), and this often leads to early-morning drinking ('eye-opener'), which relieves the symptoms.
- Tolerance—this is when increased quantities of the substance are required to produce the same effect. It is seen in alcohol-dependent persons who frequently consume more than 100 units of alcohol per week, although it may decrease in the latter stages of alcohol dependence.
- Neglect of other interests—the substance use takes primacy over other aspects of the patient's life, such as their career, family, or recreational activities.
- Reinstatement after abstinence—despite awareness of the potential harmful effects and attempts to stop, the previous pattern of substance use resumed soon after abstinence.

Withdrawal state with delirium

This state occurs when a withdrawal syndrome develops into a characteristic delirium. This is particularly important to diagnose given the life-threatening nature of a delirium.

Delirium tremens occurs around 2 days after cessation of drinking in about 5% of alcohol-dependent individuals, usually in association with a physical illness such as pneumonia. It is characterized by clouding of consciousness, disorientation, memory impairment, extreme agitation, and distressing hallucinations (in addition to the other symptoms of CNS excitation mentioned above). Characteristially, the visual hallucinations are of fleeting miniature humans or animals—Lilliputian hallucinations.

An even rarer neurological syndrome known as Wernicke's encephalopathy may occur. This is related to chronic deficiency of vitamin B1 (thiamine), which may occur in the alcohol dependent. It is characterized by impaired consciousness, disorientation, memory impairment, ataxia (broad-based gait), and ophthalmoplegia (ocular palsies, nystagmus, fixed pupils). It is thought to develop from haemorrhagic lesions within the cerebellum, thalamus, ventricular system, brainstem, and mamillary bodies.

Psychotic disorder ('drug-induced psychosis')

Psychotic disorder is the development of psychotic symptoms within 2 days of consuming the substance. It is distinct from the previous disorder and the effects of intoxication in that it occurs in clear consciousness and persists beyond the period the original substance exerts its effect. This disorder resolves spontaneously, usually within 1 month, but may at the time appear indistinguishable from an affective psychosis or schizophrenia.

Alcohol hallucinosis is a commonly described condition whereby the patient describes persistent second-person auditory hallucinations. These occur in clear consciousness (i.e. not during intoxication or withdrawal) and usually consist of simple words or phrases.

Amnesic syndrome

Alcohol-induced amnesic syndrome, or Korsakoff's psychosis, is related to vitamin B_1 deficiency and is a common sequel of Wernicke's encephalopathy.

Dementia syndrome

This presents similarly to the typical dementia syndrome described in Chapter 6, although, like the amnesic syndrome, must be clearly related to prolonged heavy use of the substance. As with the above, symptoms may persist or improve after discontinuation of the substance.

Other psychoactive substances

Problems related to the use of illegal (and, sometimes, legal) psychoactive drugs are extremely common in psychiatry, particularly among adolescents and young adults. The commonly used term 'substance abuse' is as unspecific as 'alcohol abuse'; and as with alcohol, it is useful to think in terms of the specific clinical syndromes that may be produced by the drug. Moreover, the classes of drugs described in this chapter vary enormously in their physiological effects and need to be considered individually.

The main classes of drugs, their mechanisms of action, and the specific clinical syndromes they produce are listed in Figs 7.2 and 7.3.

Amphetamine

Acute effects Dilated pupils, increased or decreased blood pressure and pulse, perspiration, agitation, euphoria, hypervigilance, and other mood changes.

Chronic effects Weight loss, tolerance, craving, and paranoid psychosis. On withdrawal, there may be

Main classes of psychoactive substances		
Drug (other names–route of administration)	**Related compounds**	**Mechanism of action**
amphetamine (oral/IV/smoked/snorted)	methamphetamine ('speed', purified form known as 'ice') dextroamphetamine ('dexy's midnight runners') methylphenidate	CNS stimulant: • inhibition of noradrenaline, dopamine, and serotonin uptake • increases release of dopamine
cocaine (smoked/snorted/inhaled/IV)	cocaine hydrochloride cocaine alkaloid (which may be prepared into the more potent 'crack')	CNS stimulant: • sympathomimetic activity • direct action on temperature regulation • local anaesthetic • increases dopamine release, blocks dopamine, noradrenaline, and serotonin reuptake
ecstasy or MDMA (methylene-dioxy-methamphetamine– oral/IV)	—	CNS stimulant: • stimulation of serotonin systems and increased dopamine release • direct action on temperature regulation
LSD (lysergic acid diethylamide–oral/IV/ smoked)	psilocybin ('magic mushrooms') mescalin	hallucinogenic that causes hyperarousal of CNS by mediation of serotonin systems
phenlycyclidine ('PCP, angel dust'– oral/smoked/IV/snorted)	ketamine	hallucinogenic that results from antagonism of the N-methyl-D-aspartate (NDMA)-PCP receptor complex
cannabis ('marijuana, hash, weed, dope, grass, skunk'– smoked/oral/IV)	—	direct action on cannabinoid receptor sites
opioids (smoked/oral/IV/snorted)	heroin methadone morphine pethidine dipipanone	direct action on opioid receptor sites (central and peripheral)
benzodiazepines (oral/IV)	temazepam especially	CNS depressant that causes potentiation of GABA (inhibitory neurotransmitter) transmission
inhalents (may be heated to increase speed of action)	huge variety of commercial products used, e.g. petrol, solvents, paints, cosmetics	similar to alcohol, initial CNS stimulation followed by CNS depression

Fig. 7.2 Main classes of psychoactive substances.

The terms 'alcoholism' and 'alcohol misuse' should be avoided; they are often loosely applied to any of the disorders described above. The syndromes described can be thought of as a 'hierarchy of severity', progressing from acute intoxication to potentially irreversible dementia.

several days of sleep disturbance, increased appetite, low mood, fatigue, and psychomotor changes.

Ecstasy is similar in effect but additionally gives rise to hyperpyrexia, dehydration, and hyponatraemia, due to direct effects on temperature regulation and antidiuretic hormone (ADH) production.

Cocaine

Acute effects Similar to those of amphetamine. Vivid hallucinations are often described, including formication (the sensation of insects crawling beneath the skin). In overdose, death may occur from hypertensive crisis or arrhythmias.

Chronic effects Nasal septum perforation or ulceration. The withdrawal syndrome is similar to amphetamine.

LSD

Acute effects Dilated pupils, tachycardia, perspiration, blurred vision, incoordination, euphoria (or depression), impaired judgement, and perceptual disturbances. 'Synaesthesia' describes blending of senses, e.g. tasting smell.

Chronic effects Tolerance and craving develop; LSD rarely causes a persistent psychosis, although flashbacks occur—these are the re-experiencing of the perceptual disturbance after use.

Cannabis

Acute effects Conjunctival injection, dry mouth, tachycardia, euphoria, relaxation, and altered time-perception and judgement.

Chronic effects Tolerance, craving, psychosis, and flashbacks can occur in heavy users; the rarely reported withdrawal syndrome consists of sleep disturbance, nausea, perspiration, and tremor.

Clinical syndromes associated with the use of psychoactive substances					
Drug	**Intoxication state**	**Dependence state**	**Withdrawal state +/- delirium**	**Psychotic disorder**	**Amnesic syndrome/dementia**
amphetamine	√	√	√	√	
cocaine	√	√	√	√	
LSD	√	√		√	
phenylcyclidine	√	√		√	
cannabis	√	√	√	√	
opioids	√	√	√	√	
benzodiazepines	√	√	√	√	√
inhalants	√	√		√	√

Fig. 7.3 Clinical syndromes associated with the use of psychoactive substances.

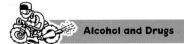

Opioids

Acute effects Conjunctival injection, constricted pupils, slurred speech, euphoria, apathy, and impaired judgement and consciousness.

Chronic effects Constipation, tolerance, and intense craving.

Withdrawal syndrome This can last for between 6 hours and 10 days. Symptoms comprise low mood, agitation, dilated pupils, vomiting, muscle pain, lacrimation, diarrhoea, cramps, fever, piloerection, gooseflesh (cold turkey), and sleep disturbance.

Overdose Pupils may dilate (anoxia), respiratory depression, hypotension, and coma.

Pregnancy Use of opioids during pregancy may lead to prematurity, low birth weight, and neonatal withdrawal (tremor, irritability, restlessness, high-pitched cry).

Benzodiazepines

Acute effects Impaired consciousness, nystagmus, disinhibition, mood changes, and perceptual disturbance.

Chronic use Effects are similar to those with alcohol in the development of tolerance, craving, and a withdrawal syndrome.

Inhalants

Acute effects Impaired consciousness, nystagmus, unsteady gait, vomiting, euphoria, disinhibition, and psychosis.

Chronic effects Weight loss, hepatorenal damage, peripheral neuropathy, arrhythmias, and bone marrow suppression; tolerance and craving occur after prolonged use.

Differential diagnosis

The variety of clinical syndromes associated with alcohol and substance misuse results in a wide differential diagnosis. This difficulty may be further compounded by the comorbid existence of another psychiatric disorder; for example, a person with a severe depressive illness may increase their alcohol consumption (resulting in dependence) to alleviate their initial depressive symptoms. It is important that a psychiatric history clarifies which came first.

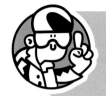

The withdrawal syndromes of alcohol/benzodiazepines and opioids are quite different—learn these well.

The following list clarifies the most common diagnostic difficulties.

Psychotic disorder (e.g. schizophrenia, delusional disorder)

Excessive alcohol consumption may directly cause alcoholic hallucinosis and is particularly related to delusions of jealousy ('Othello syndrome'). It is, however, more common for a psychosis to coincide with the misuse of illegal substances, particularly amphetamine and cocaine. Several diagnostic possibilities arise:

- The psychosis was caused by the substance.
- An underlying psychotic disorder was precipitated by the substance.
- An underlying psychotic disorder was exacerbated by the substance.
- The substance was taken after the onset of the psychotic disorder (perhaps to alleviate symptoms).
- There is no relation between the psychotic disorder and substance.

In clinical practice, the most important distinction is between the first scenario and all of the others (which assume the disorder would have occurred without using the substance). An underlying psychotic disorder is more likely if:

- Evidence of the disorder (e.g. prodromal symptoms and decline in personal functioning) occurs before the substance use.
- The disorder persists beyond (more than 1 month) and independent of the substance use.

Affective disorders

A wide variety of mood changes are seen during intoxication and withdrawal from substances. They are usually brief in duration. Most alcohol-dependent patients complain of depressed mood, caused by the CNS depressant qualities of the drug and the personal consequences that result. Furthermore, biological symptoms of depression (sleep disturbance, appetite disturbance, sexual dysfunction) are unreliable, as dependence itself causes these symptoms. Therefore, cognitive symptoms (e.g. worthlessness, hopelessness, guilt) and, in particular, suicidal ideation are the best indicators of either a primary or secondary depressive disorder.

Anxiety disorders
Excessive alcohol consumption may cause a variety of phobic, panic, and generalized-anxiety symptoms, particularly during withdrawal. Again, the anxiety disorder itself may have prompted the excessive alcohol use (as alcohol is anxiolytic); ultimately this is counterproductive because of the effects of tolerance and withdrawal.

Dementia, delirium, or amnesic syndromes secondary to other causes
These are clinically indistinguishable from their substance-induced counterparts.

Non-organic sleep disorders and sexual dysfunction
These are described in Chapter 10.

Discussion of vignette
What is Ms AD's diagnosis?
The patient was drinking in excess of 150 units of alcohol per week—this is far in excess of recommended safe limits. She described increasing consumption over a prolonged period, suggesting tolerance, and had a daily stereotyped pattern of drinking. She described physiological withdrawal symptoms on cessation of drinking (leading to early-morning drinking), a craving for alcohol, and reinstatement of drinking after abstinence. Her presentation thus supports a diagnosis of alcohol dependence. Further inquiry is needed to establish whether her depressive and anxiety symptoms are primary or secondary to this disorder; and whether her excessive alcohol use had led to the break-up of her marriage.

How are alcohol problems assessed?
Eliciting an accurate alcohol history requires tact and sensitivity because of the continuing stigmatization of alcohol problems. Many patients underestimate their levels of consumption and may present with another (alcohol-related) complaint. Important steps to follow are:

- Record the levels of consumption, establishing the number of units consumed per week. It is important to record systematically the number and type of drinks consumed throughout each day of the week, establishing a drink diary (Fig. 7.4).
- Establish whether there is underlying alcohol dependence; it is therefore crucial to ask questions along the lines of the six criteria for dependence listed earlier.
- Follow up cues in the history, such as heavy drinking within the family, sexual or sleep problems, reasons for work or financial problems, and reasons for past violence or offending behaviour.
- Consider the effect of alcohol on each of the medical, psychological, and social axes. For example: medical—acute withdrawal symptoms, blackouts during intoxication, chronic physical complaints; psychological—mood, psychotic symptoms, cognitive functioning; social—relationships, work, social activities, offending behaviour.

How are problems caused by other drugs assessed?
Problems due to other drugs are assessed using an approach similar to that used for alcohol problems, remembering that substance use is often underestimated or denied. It is important to ask about:

Assessment of alcohol intake: alcohol units

1 unit of alcohol =
1/2 pint ordinary (3%) beer
1 glass table (9%) wine
1 measure of sherry, port or spirits
(1 unit ~ 8 g alcohol)

Safe limits:
Men   <21 units/week
Women   <14 units/week (pregnancy <3 units/week)

Danger of physical harm:
Men >50 units/week
Women >35 units/week

N.B. most beers/wines consumed have a higher alcohol content than above

Fig. 7.4 Assessment of alcohol intake: alcohol units.

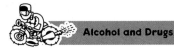

- All drugs currently and previously used (ask patients to explain any lay names mentioned). Polydrug use is common, e.g. benzodiazepines may be taken to alleviate amphetamine withdrawal.
- Chronological history of drug use—when it began, frequency of use, periods of abstinence—thereby establishing whether use is experimental (once or twice only), recreational (at weekends when socialising), or habitual (regular, irrespective of social context).
- Amounts consumed and route of administration. The former may be more accurately assessed by weekly cost.

- Medical consequences (e.g. HIV, hepatitis, local infection caused by shared needles).
- Psychological consequences (e.g. mood, concentration, perceptual disturbances).
- Social consequences (e.g. effect on relationships and peer group; debt and offending in order to finance drug use).

Relevant examination and physical investigations are detailed in Chapter 18.

A useful screening tool for dependence is the so-called CAGE questionnaire:
- **Have you ever felt you ought to <u>C</u>ut down on your drinking?**
- **Have people <u>A</u>nnoyed you by criticizing your drinking?**
- **Have you ever felt <u>G</u>uilty about your drinking?**
- **Have you ever had a drink first thing in the morning ('<u>E</u>ye-opener') to steady your nerves or treat a hangover?**

Two or more positive answers suggest a problem drinker and more extensive inquiry is needed.

8. Personality Problems

Mr PE, aged 28, is referred to psychiatric outpatients for 'anger management' advice. He describes being prone to uncontrollable outbursts of aggression, which has led to several arrests for assault. Although troubled by this problem, he believes each fight was provoked by others 'winding him up', particularly when he had had a few drinks. His short temper developed as a child. He recalls being expelled from school at the age of 15, after punching a teacher. Since leaving school he has only had a few short-term jobs, usually sacked for 'causing trouble'; and most of his relationships have ended because of his jealousy and violence.

Psychopathology

Abnormal personality development

Personality may be defined as a person's enduring pattern of relating to the environment and thinking about themselves across a wide range of personal and social contexts.

It may be broken down into a number of different traits, such as impulsiveness or stubbornness, which form the basis of personality description in psychiatry and psychology.

There is no satisfactory model of personality development, although there have been various attempts to define and categorize personality subtypes.

In Eysenck's dimensional model, for example, traits are grouped into three axes:

- Extroversion–introversion (sociability, assertiveness).
- Neuroticism–stability (anxiety, mood stability).
- Psychoticism–stability (impulsiveness, aggressiveness).

Abnormalities of personality can then be defined statistically as deviations from the population norms.

Personality develops predominantly during childhood and adolescence. It is regarded as being shaped by:

- Genetic/constitutional factors—a person's temperament.
- A person's experience and environment—e.g. deprivation, family discord, child abuse.

Personality disorders

Clinically significant deviations of 'normal' personality development are known as personality disorders.

The concept of personality disorder differs from other mental disorders in both:

- Their developmental context.
- Quantitative deviation of traits from expected norms (the symptoms of mental illness are generally regarded as qualitatively different from normal experience).

Personality disorders must have the following features:

- Marked deviations in behaviour and attitudes from the expected cultural norm.
- The abnormal behaviour and attitudes are enduring and consistent across a range of personal experiences.
- The abnormal behaviour and attitudes have their origin in childhood and adolescence.
- The disorder causes distress to the subject or to others, and creates problems in areas of personal and social functioning.

Types of personality disorder

ICD-10 defines the disorders (Figs 8.1–8.8) according to groups of related traits; they are not mutually exclusive.

DSM-IV classification includes the additional categories of:

- Narcissistic personality disorder—essentially, grandiose self-importance in both fantasy and behaviour, with a persistent need for admiration.
- Schizotypal personality disorder—similar to schizoid and paranoid personality disorders but with more prominent eccentric behaviour, overvalued ideas, and non-hallucinatory perceptual abnormalities.

Other abnormalities of personality

True personality disorders have their origin in childhood and adolescence. However, there are several situations where disorders of personality develop in adulthood:

- Organic personality disorder (see Chapter 6)—this develops secondary to a general medical cause such as encephalitis or head injury.

- Enduring personality change—this relates to an enduring personality change that occurs following either a prolonged experience where life was at risk (e.g. torture, natural disaster) or recovery from a severe mental illness.

Both of the above are characterized by more than 2 years of relative impairment in personal and social functioning and should be diagnosed only if the impairment is not due to symptoms of post-traumatic stress disorder or disorders related to the original illness (e.g. post-schizophrenia depression).

Differential diagnosis

Given the diverse forms of personality disorder, it is no surprise to find a wide differential. It is vital to exclude an underlying mental illness whenever a personality disorder is suspected, as this will have important prognostic implications.

Definition of anankastic personality disorder
preoccupation with details and rules
excessive perfectionism, single-mindedness and inflexibility in behaviour and attitudes to the extent that task completion and decision-making are impaired
excessive doubt, caution, and self-criticism
insistence that others conform to their own standards
Although intrusive thoughts or impulses may occur, the disorder is distinct from obsessive–compulsive disorder in that true obsessions and compulsions do not occur

Fig. 8.1 Definition of anankastic (obsessive–compulsive) personality disorder.

Definition of anxious (avoidant) personality disorder
preoccupation with feelings of inadequacy and inferiority
feelings of tension and apprehension
avoidance of personal relationships and social situations for fear of rejection or negative criticism
reluctance to take risks or take part in new activities

Fig. 8.2 Definition of anxious (avoidant) personality disorder.

Definition of dependent personality disorder
excessive submissiveness and subordination to others with reduced capacity to take responsibility for their own actions and make decisions
excessive fears of being abandoned by those they are dependent on, going to great lengths to engender support and reassurance from others
preoccupation with feelings of incompetence and inability to care for themselves

Fig. 8.3 Definition of dependent personality disorder.

Definition of dissocial (antisocial) personality disorder
low tolerance to frustration with tendency to react aggressively
excessive irresponsibility and rejection of social norms; tendency for impulsive, short-term gains without fear of potential consequences
others are blamed for their behaviour
inability to experience guilt or remorse
inability to form long-term relationships

Fig. 8.4 Definition of dissocial (antisocial) personality disorder.

Definition of borderline personality disorder

emotionally unstable with excessive mood fluctuation usually lasting a few hours but occasionally several days. Containing feelings of anger are particularly difficult
recurrent suicidal threats or attempts, such as overdosing or self-mutilation
other impulsive behaviour such as substance misuse or promiscuity which could be dangerous for the individual
tendency to form intense and volatile relationships
disturbance of self image with characteristic feelings of emptiness, boredom and fear of being abandoned by others

Fig. 8.5 Definition of borderline (emotionally unstable) personality disorder.

Definition of histrionic personality disorder

prone to self-dramatization particularly through activities where they are the centre of attention
emotionally shallow, suggestible, exaggerated expressions, and overconcern with their appearance
self-indulgence and manipulation of others for their own needs

Fig. 8.6 Definition of histrionic personality disorder.

Definition of paranoid personality disorder

distrust and suspiciousness of others, extreme sensitivity to criticism plus a tendency to misconstrue the remarks or actions of others
incapacity to forgive others and tendency to bear grudges
excessive sense of self-importance and personal rights

Fig. 8.7 Definition of paranoid personality disorder.

Definition of schizoid personality disorder

emotional coldness and lack of warmth displayed towards others, few activities provide pleasure
prefers to be alone, little interest in social relationships or sexual experiences
indifferent to social conventions, personal criticism
excessively introspective preferring solitary activities

Fig. 8.8 Definition of schizoid personality disorder.

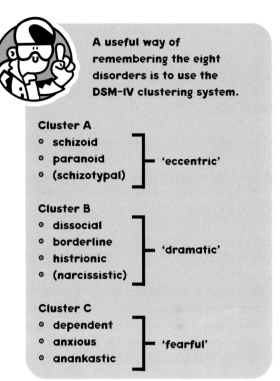

A useful way of remembering the eight disorders is to use the DSM-IV clustering system.

Cluster A
- schizoid
- paranoid
- (schizotypal) — 'eccentric'

Cluster B
- dissocial
- borderline
- histrionic
- (narcissistic) — 'dramatic'

Cluster C
- dependent
- anxious
- anankastic — 'fearful'

Dementia

The chronic personality change associated with dementia (especially frontal lobe dementia) may resemble any of the personality disorders (in particular, paranoid). However, unlike dementia, personality disorders develop in early life and are not associated with deteriorating cognitive function.

Substance Misuse Disorders

These are often closely related: the impulsive, immediate-pleasure-seeking traits of dissocial, histrionic, and borderline personality disorders frequently lead to harmful substance use. However, substance dependence itself frequently leads to personally damaging and reckless behaviour. Therefore, a comorbid personality disorder should be considered only if it developed before the damaging substance use.

Psychotic disorders

The overvalued persecutory ideas of paranoid personality disorders may resemble paranoid schizophrenia. In addition, the social withdrawal and

61

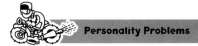

emotional flattening of schizoid personalities may resemble residual schizophrenia. However, the past or present existence of true delusions or hallucinations and a history of deterioration after normal personality development should always point towards a psychotic illness.

Affective disorders

Dissocial, borderline, and histrionic personality disorders can resemble bipolar or depressive disorders in both their behavioural manifestations and their tendency towards mood lability. The presence of psychotic symptoms, biological symptoms, and persistent mood changes (>2 weeks) should indicate an affective disorder.

Phobic and panic disorders

Both anxious and dependent personalities may be confused with phobic and panic disorders, although the latter can usually be differentiated by their:

- Deterioration from a premorbid level of functioning.
- Episodic or situation-related development of symptoms.
- Presence of intense cognitive and autonomic experiences of anxiety.

Obsessive–compulsive disorder

The excessive hoarding, attention to detail, and list-making of anankastic personalities may resemble obsessive–compulsive disorder (OCD): in fact, they rarely coexist. True obsessions and compulsions indicate OCD.

Childhood autism, Asperger's disorder and learning disability

These resemble schizoid and anankastic personalities, and are discussed in Chapter 11.

Discussion of vignette

What is Mr PE's diagnosis?

Mr PE has long-standing problems of aggression, jealousy, and oversensitivity to the remarks of others, which appear to have deleteriously affected his educational, occupational, and social performances. Such traits may represent a dissocial, paranoid, or borderline personality disorder. However, it must be stressed that his problems may be secondary to another disorder—e.g. related to alcohol or drug

intoxication, schizophrenia (ideas of jealousy and persecution may be delusional), or a mood disorder (irritability may occur in depression and mania). Ultimately, diagnosis of a personality disorder as the sole cause of his presentation is dependent on carefully excluding other disorders first.

How is personality assessed?

Assessment of personality is one of the most difficult and underrated parts of the psychiatric examination. 'Premorbid personality' refers to the patient's usual personality before the onset of mental illness or presenting problem; it is typically questioned towards the end of a psychiatric history. Much of a person's personality can be judged objectively from other parts of the history.

Objective measures of personality are:

- Educational attainment and behaviour at school.
- Work history.
- Forensic history.
- Sexual and social relationships.
- Interests and activities.

Persistent problems or instability in any of these areas may point towards abnormal personality development. Childhood conduct disorder (see Chapter 11) often precedes adult dissocial personality disorder.

 Patients rarely present with a 'personality problem'. Personality disorders usually present to psychiatrists:

- Comorbidly with another disorder, e.g. substance related, psychotic disorder, mood disorder.
- At times of 'crisis', when inadequate coping mechanisms are overwhelmed, e.g. relationship difficulties, unemployment.
- Following deliberate self-harm (the lifetime suicide risk for personality disorders is around 10%).

Direct inquiry into the patient's subjective assessment of their personality is then sought. For example, an opening question could be: 'I realize this is a difficult question, but how would you and others describe your previous personality and character?' As this is indeed a difficult question, infuriatingly, most people respond: 'Happy-go-lucky'! Rather than moving on to the next part of the history, it is preferable to try and question specific areas of personality function. To avoid trapping patients by over-closed questions, the various traits of personality can be tested by offering a number of scenarios, e.g. 'Before your illness...'

- 'Were you prone to mood swings or did people see you as a generally happy person?' (mood stability).
- 'If your boss criticized your work and told you to start again using his method, how would you react?' (reaction to criticism).
- 'Would you have felt uneasy if alone in a busy supermarket or in a pub, or if you were asked to give a speech?' (self confidence, using progressively more threatening situations).
- 'Did you prefer your own company, or the company of others?' (sociability).
- 'What sort of situations would make you so angry that you would lose your temper?' (anger management).

The above questions are merely suggestions; it is important to devise your own scheme. Also, remember to follow up any cues in the patient's answers—why are they unable to make any friends?

To clarify further whether there are underlying personality problems, it is important to:
- Re-interview the patient.
- Obtain a corroborative history from someone who has known the patient since childhood or adolescence.

An algorithm for personality disorders is shown in Fig. 8.9.

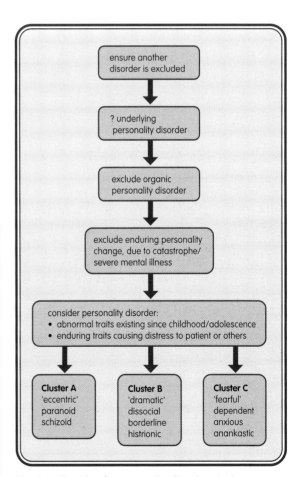

Fig. 8.9 Algorithm for personality disorders. In the hierarchy of diagnoses, personality disorders are always superseded by other disorders.

Be wary of diagnosing personality disorders, particularly in an exam situation where a corroborative history cannot be sought. The diagnosis can often be used as a derogatory label for patients we do not like or who do not get better; in an exam it is better to tentatively postulate abnormal traits that require further exploration. Furthermore, there is often considerable overlap between the diagnostic categories (e.g. dissocial and borderline traits)—patients do not fit into neat boxes!

9. Physical Complaints and Underlying Mental Illness

THE PATIENT WITH PHYSICAL COMPLAINTS AND UNDERLYING MENTAL ILLNESS

Mr PC, a busy taxi-driver aged 32, has consulted his family doctor more than 20 times in the last 3 years. He has no history of mental health problems, but over this time has presented with a variety of physical symptoms, including back and knee pain, throat discomfort with regurgitation of food, persistent nausea, abdominal pain, and loose stools. The family doctor has performed numerous physical examinations but has found nothing remarkable, and various blood tests, all of which have been normal. When Mr PC was referred to the rheumatologists, no abnormality was found in his knee or back; X-rays and antibody titres being normal. The gastroenterologists produced further negative results despite complex investigations including a barium swallow. The list of complaints has recently been augmented by episodes of tingling in his hands, and Mr PC has been referred to psychiatry outpatients. He explains that although none of the symptoms stop him driving his taxi or engaging in social activities, he finds the pains and nausea unbearable and is sure that the medics are missing something. He is angry with his family doctor, who rejected the need for a further detailed scan of his knee, and plans instead to consult an osteopath privately.

Psychopathology

Somatization and somatic symptoms

Somatization is the generation of recurrent physical symptoms—referred to as 'somatic symptoms'. It is associated with a demand for medical investigation in case the symptoms are harbingers of an underlying physical illness.

Multiple symptoms may be experienced, involving different systems and areas of the body. Gastrointestinal, cardiovascular, genitourinary, and locomotor symptoms may occur, including pain and unpleasant sensations like nausea, bloatedness, loose bowel motions, and genital discomfort. Skin rash and the neurological symptoms of paraesthesia and numbness may also be part of the syndrome. Alternatively, the symptoms may be exclusively those of autonomic arousal or may solely involve the experience of pain.

Hypochondriasis

Hypochondriasis involves preoccupation with the idea of having a specific serious physical illness, or of having a deformity or disfigurement, in the absence of evidence that this is actually the case. The

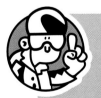

A 'somatic syndrome' is also described in depression. This term refers to the biological symptoms of depression (see Chapter 1) and is not the same as the somatic symptoms discussed here.

preoccupation is fuelled by the presence of a physical sign or symptom which the patient interprets as being indicative of a greater underlying problem. The preoccupation is not so strong as to be delusional—the patient is aware that their fear could be out of proportion with the signs or symptoms—but it persists despite medical reassurance that nothing is seriously amiss.

Conversion

Conversion is the production of a physical symptom in response to an acute psychological stress. The DSM-IV and ICD-10 classifications have handled 'conversion disorders' in slightly different ways, although in both cases the definitions are built upon the precept that they involve a 'conversion' of a stress in the mind to a symptom in the body.

DSM-IV limits conversion phenomena to those that manifest as a single neurological symptom, including:
- Paraesthesia (tingling sensations).
- Numbness.
- Abnormal gait.
- Other movement disturbance.

And more dramatic manifestations such as:
- Paralysis.
- Seizures.
- Blindness.
- Mutism.

In contrast, ICD-10 merges conversion with dissociative disorders, including dissociative amnesia, fugue, and stupor (see Chapter 4), as well as with the less complex neurological deficits found in the DSM-IV conversion category.

Differential diagnosis

Somatoform disorders

Somatization disorder

Features of somatization disorder include:
- Two years or more of a range of variable symptoms which are recurrent and cannot be explained by detectable physical disorders.
- Preoccupation with the symptoms causes distress and leads to the patient demanding three or more sets of investigations or specialist referrals, but, despite this, the patient still refuses to be reassured that nothing is medically wrong.

- At least six of the symptoms listed in Fig. 9.1 are present.

Persistent somatoform pain disorder

In persistent somatoform pain disorder, somatic symptoms are confined to pain, which may occur in various diverse regions of the body and which must be severe and distressing for at least 6 months.

Somatoform autonomic dysfunction

In somatoform autonomic dysfunction, although the patient attributes their symptoms to a disorder of the cardiovascular, gastrointestinal, respiratory, or genitourinary system, there is no evidence of true pathological changes affecting the relevant organ system. There must be two symptoms typical of autonomic arousal (palpitations, sweating, flushing, dry mouth, or abdominal churning) and a further non-specific symptom referred to the relevant organ system (e.g. chest pain or precordial discomfort).

Hypochondriacal disorder

For a diagnosis of hypochondriacal disorder there must be:
- A persistent belief lasting 6 months or more that the individual has one or two serious physical diseases, one of which must be named.

Somatic symptoms, arranged by body system	
Body system	**Symptom**
gastrointestinal	abdominal pain nausea bloatedness bad taste in mouth food vomited or regurgitated frequent/loose motions
cardiovascular	breathlessness without exertion chest pain
genitourinary	dysuria or frequency of micturition unpleasant genital sensations increased or changed vaginal discharge
neurological	joint/limb pain numbness/tingling
skin	skin discoloration skin rash

Fig. 9.1 Somatic symptoms, arranged by body system.

- Evidence of distress or impairment in functioning caused by the belief or by the symptoms associated with the 'disease', leading to the seeking of medical attention.
- Persistent refusal to accept medical reassurance as to the lack of a physical cause for the symptoms, for more than brief periods.

Dysmorphophobia (body dysmorphic disorder) is a related condition involving a persistent belief of deformity or disfigurement, again causing distress and producing a demand for medical input.

Make sure you remember that malingering is distinguished from factitious disorder through the presence of a conscious external motivating factor. In factitious disorder there is no evidence of such a factor beyond the wish to be a patient or take on the 'sick role'.

Conversion disorder (DSM-IV)
In the DSM-IV conversion disorder:
- A symptom (e.g. paraesthesia, abnormal gait) occurs which is suggestive of a neurological or other general medical condition but is associated directly with a psychological conflict or stress.
- It cannot be explained by any medical condition or substance (after appropriate investigation), nor is it produced deliberately or feigned (as in factitious disorder or malingering).
- The symptom causes distress or impairment in functioning, or evokes a need for medical attention.

Factitious disorder and malingering
In both factitious disorder and malingering, there is repeated feigning of symptoms (including 'physical' symptoms such as abdominal pain, seizures, or fever, or 'psychiatric' symptoms such as low mood or auditory hallucinations).

Whereas in malingering the motivation for such action is clear (e.g. to avoid military action or appearance in court), in factitious disorder it may be obscure or subconscious, with no identifiable external incentive. Munchausen's syndrome is a form of factitious disorder.

No other physical or psychiatric disorder that might account for the behaviour is present.

Other psychiatric differentials
Generalized anxiety disorder and panic disorder
Symptoms of generalized anxiety disorder or panic disorder may be similar to those seen in somatoform autonomic disorder; however, anxiety or panic attacks and the psychosocial factors that provoke them are seen by the patient as the problem, rather than an underlying physical illness (see Chapter 2).

Depressive disorder
Physical symptoms are often provoked by depression. When symptoms have clearly occurred secondarily to or as part of a depressive episode, somatoform disorders are not usually diagnosed. Certain characteristic symptoms such as poor appetite, weight loss, early-morning wakening, and loss of libido are so common in depression (see Chapter 1) that ICD-10 includes the category 'depressive episode with somatic syndrome'—but note that these symptoms are not the same as those typical of somatization disorder .

Schizophrenia
Again, somatoform disorders are not diagnosed when the symptoms are secondary to schizophrenia (see Chapter 5). Note that hypochondriachal ideas may be held with delusional intensity and somatic symptoms may have a delusional interpretation (e.g. caused by aliens), so it is essential to look for underlying psychotic disorders.

Discussion of vignette
Mr PC has long-standing problems with a number of recurrent physical symptoms. They first arrived in his late twenties and have persisted over the past 3 years.

Could the physical symptoms be due to an undiagnosed general medical condition?
Given the number of different body systems which the symptoms now cover—locomotor, gastrointestinal, and, lately, neurological—they could be explained only by a multisystem disease such as systemic lupus erythematosus, thyroid problems, or multiple sclerosis.

However, Mr PC has already had the attention of his family doctor, who has performed numerous laboratory tests, and then further investigation by a rheumatologist and by a gastroenterologist. The odds are now firmly against there being an undiagnosed multisystem disease.

Somatization or hypochondriasis?

Although Mr PC refuses to accept medical reassurance, we can rule out hypochondriasis immediately: although Mr PC presents with a variety of symptoms, he is not preoccupied by one or more named diseases, nor is he worried about deformity or disfigurement.

The picture is more typical of somatization. Mr PC fulfils the ICD-10 criteria for somatization disorder in that his symptoms are multiple and variable, have lasted at least 2 years, and are not explained by detectable physical disorders. Furthermore, the symptoms have bothered Mr PC sufficiently that he has repeatedly sought medical contact with a number of doctors but he is still unimpressed by assurances that there is nothing physically wrong.

To justify an ICD-10 diagnosis of somatization disorder, Mr PC must have at least six of the symptoms listed in Fig. 9.1: he reaches this threshold. Careful questioning may reveal further appropriate symptoms, but the temptation to put closed questions to a person crying out to have his or her problems taken seriously—and thus generating false information—must be avoided. Note that Mr PC might fall beneath the threshold for a DSM-IV diagnosis of somatization disorder, where the somewhat stricter criteria require not only that the symptoms begin before the age of 30 but also that they cover each of four categories (pain, gastrointestinal, sexual, and pseudoneurological symptoms).

Considering the episodes of tingling in Mr PC's hands (paraesthesias), would a diagnosis of the DSM-IV conversion disorder be appropriate?

Although this is an apparently neurological symptom occurring at a time when there is already psychological distress (i.e. the distress caused by other symptoms), it is more appropriate to consider the paraesthesias as part and parcel of the existing somatization or somatoform disorder. Conversion disorder normally refers to an acute onset of a single neurological symptom (which may be as dramatic as limb paralysis or blindness).

What about factitious disorder and malingering?

If we suspected that Mr PC had engineered his complaints for an obvious gain—to attract financial rewards or achieve an easier lifestyle—we would consider malingering. If we thought his symptoms were deliberately manufactured but were without motivation, factitious disorder would be considered. Given that Mr PC has faithfully continued to drive his taxi in spite of his symptoms and is prepared to spend his own money on further investigation, it is unlikely that such diagnoses are relevant here.

Other psychiatric diagnoses?

Although a full mental-state examination is required, there is nothing in Mr PC's story to suggest that schizophrenia or depression is a primary cause of the symptoms. There is no evidence of free-floating anxiety or discrete spontaneous panic attacks which might point to diagnoses of generalized anxiety disorder or panic disorder.

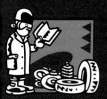

10. Problems of Physiological Function

THE PATIENT WITH EATING PROBLEMS

Miss EP is 18 years old and has recently left school having succeeded in her exams, obtaining a place at a leading university. Her mother finally persuaded her to see the family doctor to discuss her weight and eating habits, now that her exams are over—she had hitherto insisted vehemently that there was nothing to discuss. The doctor notes that for her height of 157 cm she weighs only 42 kg. Miss EP's mother points out that a year ago her daughter weighed over 57 kg but has appeared to lose weight progressively since the autumn term. Miss EP insists she eats reasonably and says she takes regular exercise—especially jogging and gymnasium work. When asked whether she is ever sick after a meal, she refuses to answer, staring with apparent indignation at the question. On physical examination the doctor notes that Miss EP appears very thin, her arms so narrow that her muscles appear almost wasted. Miss EP is impatient throughout, stressing that nothing is wrong and annoyed at being kept from her university preparations.

Psychopathology

Weight change

The body mass index (BMI) is a simple way of assessing whether a patient is underweight, normal, overweight, or obese. The weight in kilograms is divided by the square of the height in metres. The recommended BMI is 20–25 kg/m^2, with 25–30 kg/m^2 indicating an overweight subject and values greater than 30 kg/m^2 indicating obesity. Values below 20 kg/m^2 are associated with being underweight. In anorexia nervosa, weight loss down to 15% or more below the norm—reflected in a BMI value of below 17 kg/m^2—occurs.

Numerous physiological changes may be associated with weight loss. These include:
- Cachexia (loss of fat and muscle mass, decreased thyroid metabolism).
- Lanugo (development of fine hair over most of the body).
- Hormonal change involving disruption of the hypothalamic–pituitary–gonadal axis. In females this

may cause reductions in luteinizing hormone (LH) and follicle-stimulating hormone (FSH), producing amenorrhoea (cessation of periods) or irregularities of the menstrual cycle. In males there may be loss of sexual interest and potency. In younger patients, puberty—and in particular the development of secondary sexual characteristics—may be delayed.
- Osteoporosis.
- Cardiac arrhythmias.
- Hypercholesterolaemia.

Distorted body image

Classically, patients with anorexia nervosa and bulimia nervosa believe they are too fat and develop an enveloping fear of fatness: they aim to reach an ideal weight that is considerably lower than that recommended for their height. Their image of their own body appears distorted in that a weight which would generally be considered very low may be seen as ideal or, possibly, still too heavy.

Strategies of moderating weight

Aside from the more conventional strategy of reducing caloric intake by avoiding foods with any more than a minimal fat content, there are a number of means by which patients concerned about their weight may seek to moderate it. Strategies include engaging in excessive exercise, self-induced vomiting after meals, and the use of purgatives, appetite suppressants, and diuretics.

In some patients, particularly those with bulimic illnesses, the picture is further complicated by bouts of excessive overeating and compulsion to eat. Such behaviour may be counteracted by the strategies suggested above, and even by imposing periods of starvation between times of binge eating.

Differential diagnosis
Anorexia nervosa
An ICD-10 diagnosis of anorexia nervosa requires:

- Weight loss to 15% below normal weight for age and height (in adults this means a body mass index of 17 kg/m^2 or less), this being self-induced by avoidance of 'fattening' foods.
- Perception of being too fat (even though underweight) and dread of fatness, associated with the pursuit of an abnormally low 'target' weight.
- Evidence of endocrine disturbance (amenorrhoea in females and loss of sexual interest and potency in males).
- Absence of the bulimic symptoms of overeating bouts and craving food.

Activities such as self-induced vomiting and use of laxatives may occur in anorexia nervosa but are not essential to make the diagnosis.

Bulimia nervosa
An ICD-10 diagnosis of bulimia nervosa requires:
- Recurrent bouts of overeating.

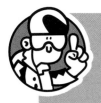
There is one exception to the above diagnostic criteria—women on an oral contraceptive may still experience vaginal bleeding.

- Persistent preoccupation with eating and a craving for food.
- Fattening effects of food counteracted by one or more of the following: self-induced vomiting, self-induced purging, intermittent starvation, use of drugs (appetite suppressants, thyroid preparations, diuretics).

Bulimic patients need not be underweight and, unlike in anorexia nervosa, do not need to have a body mass index below a certain threshold before the diagnosis can be made. In fact, the majority of bulimic patients have a body mass index within the normal range.

In contrast, the DSM-IV classification recognizes that patients with anorexia nervosa may indulge in binges and describes 'anorexia nervosa, binge eating type' for those who have the classical severe weight loss, fear of fatness, distorted body image, and endocrine changes, as well as episodes of losing control over eating and consuming amounts of food which most people would consider excessive.

Atypical anorexia and atypical bulimia
Diagnoses of atypical anorexia and atypical bulimia may be applied to patients who fulfil most but not all of the above criteria. For example, a patient who lacks the perception of being too fat and a dread of fatness but has all the other features of anorexia nervosa could be considered to have atypical anorexia.

Organic causes of low weight
The possibility of weight loss being due to an underlying organic disorder should always be considered, especially when it appears that no weight-reducing strategies are consciously being used.

The following diseases may cause weight loss:
- Malignancies.
- Addison's disease.
- Inflammatory bowel disease (Crohn's disease, ulcerative colitis).
- Malabsorption.

- Diabetes mellitus.
- Hyperthyroidism.

Other psychiatric differentials
Depressive disorders and bipolar affective disorder
Although some depressed patients may put on weight through 'comfort eating', others experience marked loss of appetite and may experience significant weight loss. Patients with anorexia nervosa, by contrast, retain their appetite until the late stages of the disease and remain interested in food-related items like recipes. Depression may coexist with an eating disorder, in which case both conditions should be diagnosed and treated (see Chapter 1).

Abuse of alcohol or illicit substances
Diet often suffers in the presence of substance abuse (see Chapter 7).

Psychotic disorders
A schizophrenic patient may have a delusion that their food is routinely poisoned by the kitchen staff and may therefore eat very little (see Chapter 5).

Obsessive–compulsive disorder
The preoccupation with body image and strife for weight loss seen in anorexia nervosa may appear similar to the obsessional thoughts and compulsive acts of obsessive–compulsive disorder (OCD): however, unlike the case in OCD, these features are not recognized as unreasonable. Although a patient with OCD may suffer weight loss when time-consuming obsessions and compulsions preclude an adequate diet (see the vignette in Chapter 3), these features are not focused on body image or food and are not directly self-induced—hence, an eating disorder cannot be diagnosed.

Discussion of vignette
Miss EP has attended her doctor with great reluctance, as is often the case with patients suffering from eating disorders. Her refusal to divulge more than a few basic facts makes the diagnosis as yet unclear.

What evidence is there to suggest Miss EP may have an eating disorder?
Significant weight loss
Assuming her mother's assertion that she weighed over 57 kg last year is correct, Miss EP has lost at least 15 kg, representing at least 20–25% of her original body weight and producing a BMI of 17 kg/m^2—sufficiently underweight for a diagnosis of anorexia nervosa to be considered. There is also some evidence of physical changes, including loss of muscle mass.

A suggestion of distorted body image
The consultation was terminated by Miss EP insisting that 'nothing was wrong' with her weight. While this may have simply reflected an impatience with having to attend in the first place, taken literally it indicates a belief that her low weight is fine, pointing towards the presence of an eating disorder. Her real view may be that at 42 kg she is still too fat, and perhaps further weight loss may be planned.

Use of a further strategy to prevent weight gain
Even if Miss EP were ingesting an adequate number of calories per day, she may have counteracted this by use of strategies to stop their absorption or to use them up quickly. She has admitted to regular exercise and it would be necessary to quantify just how much jogging and gymnasium work she does each week. An empathic clinician may also be able to elicit whether she undertakes self-induced vomiting or has used any medications to prevent weight gain.

What do we need to know to be sure she has an eating disorder?
To confirm the diagnosis of an eating disorder, we need to know more about Miss EP's attitude about her present weight and to decide whether she indeed has the distortion of body image and fear of fatness characteristic in both anorexia nervosa and bulimia nervosa.

Miss EP has intimated that she believes she eats reasonably, despite her marked weight loss. It would be useful to confirm this with her mother, as Miss EP's idea of 'reasonable' may be significantly less than the norm. She may take regular meals but, through fear of gaining weight, eat very small portions or restrict herself to foods with the bare minimum of calories.

An alternative explanation for weight loss should always be actively sought, by considering the medical conditions and psychiatric disorders listed above. If closer questioning revealed no real distorted body image nor fear of fatness, it would be especially relevant to ascertain whether Miss EP's weight loss was secondary to major depression associated with loss of appetite, to abuse of an illicit substance, or to an undiagnosed medical condition.

71

How would we establish whether the eating disorder was anorexia nervosa or bulimia nervosa?

Assume now that we confirmed that Miss EP considered her present weight of 42 kg was still too high and that she had a genuine dread of appearing to be fat.

To make a firm diagnosis of anorexia nervosa, hormonal change such as amenorrhea should be present. Note that, despite their weight loss, patients with anorexia nervosa usually retain a great interest in the subject of food (e.g. in low-calorie recipes).

Given the severe weight loss a diagnosis of bulimia nervosa is unlikely. However, if it emerged that Miss EP did regularly lose control of her eating and consume amounts of food which the majority of people would consider excessive, she may be considered to have anorexia nervosa, binge eating type. Clinicians strictly observing the rules of the ICD-10 classification would probably describe such a case as anorexia nervosa complicated by bulimic symptoms.

THE PATIENT WITH SLEEP PROBLEMS

Mr SP, aged 47, has been referred to a specialist in sleep disorders by his family doctor. He is an accountant and commutes to town by train each day from his home in the outer suburbs. He sleeps restlessly and complains of tiredness and irritability at work and admits to taking an occasional nap in his office when the opportunity presents. He is particularly embarrassed to report that several times in the last 4 months he has boarded his train homeward after leaving work, only to emerge from a deep sleep 70 miles away at a seaside terminus. He relates that his job is demanding and he has a tendency to overeat—he has put on 25 kg over the last 2 years. His wife has told him to mention that his collar size has increased by two inches over the last year and that he has recently been snoring very heavily.

Psychopathology
Normal sleep
Sleep is a regular, recurrent state of quiescence in which the threshold for responding to external stimuli is much higher than in the wakeful state. Based on waves detected by the electroencephalogram (EEG), sleep can be subdivided into five characteristic stages: stages I–IV of non-rapid eye movement sleep, ranked in order of increased depth and by characteristics of the waveform, and rapid eye movement (REM) sleep, which is associated with dreaming and is more similar physiologically to the wakeful state. Normal sleep involves passing from stage I to deeper stages,

returning to stage I and to REM at intervals of 60–90 minutes. A small number of brief arousals usually occur even in the most regular and refreshing sleep, but most are not subsequently recalled.

Insomnia
Insomnia refers to a persistent difficulty in obtaining sleep of sufficient duration or quality. The problem may involve:
- Difficulty initiating sleep.
- Recurrently waking soon after getting to sleep.
- Early final waking.
- Sleep that is adequate in its duration but unsatisfactory because it is unrefreshing.

Hypersomnia

Hypersomnia refers to excessive amounts of sleeping (nocturnal sleep or daytime somnolence) or to sleep attacks, except when these features are directly due to an overall lack of sleep. The term can also be used to describe an abnormally lengthy transition from sleep to full alertness on waking.

Other sleep problems

Patients may complain of problems with their sleep–wake schedule (e.g. achieving sleep only in the daytime when night-time sleep is desired), and of nightmares (REM sleep) or sleep terrors (non-REM sleep).

Differential diagnosis

Sleep problems may be:
- Primary (e.g. non-organic insomnia).
- Secondary to psychiatric conditions or to organic or medical conditions.

Primary sleep problems

Non-organic insomnia

A diagnosis of non-organic insomnia requires:
- Insomnia at least three times a week for a month.
- Distress or interference with functioning.
- Absence of an organic or substance-related cause.

Non-organic hypersomnia

A diagnosis of non-organic hypersomnia requires:
- Hypersomnia nearly every day for a month (or less if every day).
- Distress or interference with functioning.
- Absence of an organic or substance-related cause and absence of evidence of sleep apnoea or narcolepsy.

Narcolepsy

The DSM-IV definition of narcolepsy involves:
- Irresistible sleep attacks occurring daily over 3 months which provide refreshing sleep.
- Cataplexy (sudden loss of muscle tone) or recurrent features of REM sleep (such as hypnogogic/hypnopompic hallucinations or sleep paralysis) intruding on the transition between sleep and wakefulness.
- Absence of a medical or substance-related cause.

Sleep apnoea

In the sleep apnoea syndrome, airflow is blocked at the nose or mouth, causing 'apnoeic periods' lasting 10 seconds or more and often followed by a brief arousal. When there are many such arousals (e.g. more than 30 per night), the refreshing quality of sleep is greatly diminished and patients may experience daytime tiredness and sleep attacks. For anatomical reasons, it is most likely to occur in the obese.

Sleep problems secondary to psychiatric disorders, substance-related causes, or organic disorders

Psychiatric, substance-related, and general medical causes of insomnia and hypersomnia are summarized in Fig. 10.1

Discussion of vignette

What are the areas to assess in a patient complaining of sleep problems?

The areas to assess in patients complaining of sleep problems are:
- Pattern of sleep.
- Daytime sleep.
- 'Sleep hygiene' (see below).
- Presence of medical or psychiatric disorders or other provoking factors which may interfere with sleep.

A collateral history from a 'sleep partner' may be invaluable as it is notoriously difficult to quantify your own sleep. They may also provide information on sleep hygiene, snoring, and disrupted breathing.

What questions could be asked to gain further insight into Mr SP's sleep pattern?

The following questions may be used to explore sleep pattern with a view to assessing for insomnia:
- 'What time do you go to bed and at what time do you aim to get up?'

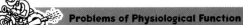

- 'Can you get to sleep quickly or do you find yourself tossing and turning for minutes or hours before dropping off?'
- 'Do you wake up repeatedly in the night or can you sleep through once you have managed to drop off ?'
- 'Do you find there is a certain hour after which it is impossible to regain sleep?

- Is the sleep refreshing or do you still feel tired in the morning?'

In some patients, hypersomnia is a more pertinent issue. Questions to ask include:
- 'Do you take naps during the day?'
- 'Do you ever suddenly or unintentionally fall asleep in the daytime?'

Summary of psychiatric, substance-related, and general medical causes of insomnia and hypersomnia			
Causes	**Insomnia**	**Hypersomnia**	**Explanation**
affective disorders			
depressive episodes	√	√	poor sleep and early morning wakening are biological symptoms of depression. Recurrent thoughts of guilt or failure make getting to sleep difficult. Lethargy and poor motivation may lead to excess sleep
hypomanic/manic episodes	√		an inexhaustible energy supply may make the sleep pattern erratic and the amount of sleep may be much reduced. When energy runs low towards the end of an episode, a patient may complain strongly of lacking sleep
anxiety disorders			
generalized anxiety disorder	√		persistent worrying prevents the sufferer from getting to sleep
panic disorder	√		nocturnal panic attacks may occur on waking
psychotic disorders			
schizophrenia	√	√	recurrent auditory hallucinations or delusions of persecution may disturb sleep. Antipsychotic drugs may cause excess sedation
substance-related			
drug effects	√	√	drugs with sedative side effects e.g. some tricyclic antidepressants, antihistamines promote sleep but may cause daytime somnolence. Other drugs have stimulant properties (e.g. caffeine, SSRIs) and may initially cause sleep disturbance
alcohol use	√	√	alcohol is a CNS depressant, promoting somnolence and is particularly associated with difficulty in getting up the next day. Alcohol dependence is associated with insomnia
drug/alcohol withdrawal	√	√	alcohol, nicotine, benzodiazepines, neuroleptics and many illicit drugs are associated with withdrawal syndromes which may produce insomnia or hypersomnia
general medical causes			
chronic pain	√		painful conditions may make it difficult to both initiate and maintain sleep
infections, neoplasia	√		associated with difficulty in maintaining sleep
endocrine and metabolic conditions	√	√	may disrupt sleep but can cause sedation and hypersomnia if blood levels of a sedating substance are raised

Fig. 10.1 Summary of psychiatric, substance-related, and general medical causes of insomnia and hypersomnia.

What questions about 'sleep hygiene' enable us to determine whether Mr SP has a suitable environment for sleeping?

Relevant questions about 'sleep hygiene' include:

- Is the bedroom quiet? Is the bed comfortable?
- Is the bedroom used for many daytime activities, so undermining its importance as a place to sleep?
- Does the patient have any regular routine before sleeping—e.g. getting washed or having a hot drink? (A regular sleep 'cue' is often helpful in promoting sleep.)

What is Mr SP's likely diagnosis?

Mr SP exhibits restless sleep and appears to make up for this both through intentional daytime napping and through dramatic sleep attacks in which sleep is so deep that he is neither roused by the stopping and starting of the train nor by the slamming of doors.

It is clearly essential to look closely for medical, psychiatric, and substance-related conditions that may interfere with sleep. For instance, chronic back pain, depression, or heavy alcohol use may all prevent sleep, and the sleep problem could be secondary to any of these. However, the best clues to the diagnosis are his rapid increase in weight, expanding collar size, and the heavy snoring observed by his wife. These features are typical of sleep apnoea.

Weight gain and increased collar size may provoke sleep apnoea by causing anatomical changes. In addition to the heavy snoring, Mr SP's wife may also have noticed the apnoeic periods where her husband appears to stop breathing—underlining the importance of taking a history from the sleep partner. When sleep apnoea is severe, there may be many apnoeic episodes and—unbeknown to the patient— very little normal sleep, leading to daytime sleep, both intentional and unexpected.

DISORDERS OF REPRODUCTION

In this section, special emphasis will be given to disorders associated with the puerperal period. However, we will start by considering problems associated with other stages of the reproductive cycle.

Menstruation

Psychological and physical symptoms are common in the few days up to the onset of menstruation. Premenstrual tension typically consists of low mood, anxiety, irritability, breast tenderness, headache, bloating, and low energy. Its cyclical nature and resolution post menstruation should avoid confusion with mood or anxiety disorders.

Menopause

Although psychological symptoms may accompany the physical changes occurring at the menopause, a relationship between the menopause and specific psychiatric disorders has not been defined.

Pregnancy

Except where the woman has had a previous psychiatric disorder, pregnancy itself does not appear to result in an increased risk of mental disorder. Symptoms that do occur tend to arise in the first or third trimester.

There are two rare pregnancy-associated conditions:

- Pseudocyesis—this is where a woman (or man) falsely believes they are pregnant, often developing symptoms of abdominal distension or amenorrhoea. The symptom may be part of a conversion disorder or psychotic disorder.
- Couvade syndrome—this is where the male partner of a pregnant woman develops the symptoms of pregnancy, such as nausea or morning sickness. The symptoms probably reflect conversion of the man's anxieties about the pregnancy into somatic symptoms.

Puerperium

Three conditions are recognized in the puerperium:

- 'Baby blues'.
- Postnatal depression.
- Puerperal psychosis.

'Baby blues'

'Baby blues' is the occurrence of mood lability, tearfulness, irritability, and a subjective feeling of 'confusion' in the first few days postpartum. It occurs to some degree in most women, spontaneously resolving on the third or fourth day postpartum.

Postnatal depression

Postnatal depression is the occurrence of mild to moderate depressive disorders in the year after childbirth and develops in approximately 10% of women. Although indistinguishable from depressive disorders in general, less emphasis should be given to somatic symptoms because sleep disturbance, energy changes, and changes in libido occur normally at this time. Unfortunately, it is a diagnosis easily missed. Warning signs include increased tearfulness, excessive concern over the baby's health, and concern at being a 'bad' mother.

Puerperal psychosis

Although puerperal psychosis is much rarer than the previous two conditions, it has the most serious consequences. This disorder occurs in approximately 0.1% of women in the year after childbirth with incidence peaking in the first two weeks postpartum. Characteristically, there is a rapid onset of psychotic symptoms which may be indistinguishable from a manic, depressive, or schizophreniform psychosis. The symptoms may vary markedly in their nature and intensity over a short space of time. Sometimes, disorientation and other signs of clouding of consciousness occur, in which case it is important to exclude the delirium of a postnatal sepsis.

Puerperal psychoses result in a greatly increased risk of suicide and infanticide (when a mentally disordered mother kills her child in the year postpartum). Questioning should include special emphasis on:

- **Suicidal ideation.**
- **Ideas of hopelessness, particularly if the mother considers the world an unfit place to raise a child.**
- **Delusions of guilt, persecution, and misidentification (believing the baby is not their own, or has been replaced by someone else).**
- **Command hallucinations instructing the mother to kill her baby.**

DISORDERS OF SEXUALITY AND GENDER

Disorders of sexuality and gender constitute a heterogenous group. Both ICD-10 and DSM-IV break down this group into three distinct types of disorder:

- Sexual dysfunction.
- Disorders of sexual preference.
- Gender identity disorders.

Sexual dysfunction

Disorders in the category 'sexual dysfunction' are concerned with difficulties a person may have participating in and in enjoying a sexual relationship. Although they are commonly complaints of physiological dysfunction, these disorders are considered as having a psychological rather than an organic origin. In clinical practice they are usually encountered as secondary to another psychiatric disorder or to the effects of prescribed psychotropic drugs.

It is useful to think of these disorders in terms of the first three stages of the sexual response cycle:

- Desire.
- Excitement.
- Orgasm.

Desire

Problems with desire can take one of two forms:

- The drive and appetite for sexual activity (libido) is reduced or completely lost.
- Sexual activity itself is actively avoided owing to resultant feelings of fear, anxiety, or disgust (sexual aversion).

Excitement

In males with problems of excitement, there is failure to achieve or maintain an erection. Unlike erectile dysfunction secondary to drug or organic causes, it is usually specific to certain situations, and masturbation erections are unimpaired. In females there is failure to achieve sufficient arousal to complete sexual activity (vasocongestion in the pelvis, vaginal lubrication, and swelling of external genitalia). These disorders are known as 'failure of genital response'.

Orgasm

Orgasm may be delayed or may fail to occur at all. Conversely, men may suffer premature ejaculation to the extent that sexual enjoyment for both partners is greatly impaired. This may in turn lead to sexual aversion. Intercourse itself may be painful for both partners (dyspareunia), and females may be specifically affected by vaginismus, where spasm of muscles surrounding the vagina prevents penile entry or causes it to be painful.

Differential diagnosis

The patient presenting with a sexual dysfunction must be carefully assessed for any evidence of underlying medical or drug-related causes (Figs. 10.2 and 10.3). In addition, there are a wide variety of psychiatric disorders that affect sexual desire and performance— notably, depressive disorders, anxiety disorders, and anorexia nervosa. This situation is further complicated by the effects of psychotropic drugs (see Chapter 15) used to treat these disorders—most of which affect sexual function.

Disorders of sexual preference (paraphilias)

The category 'disorders of sexual preference' includes those individuals who have persistent sexual desire for, and sexual behaviour towards, either non-human objects, children, or other non-consenting adults. It also includes fantasies and behaviour involving extreme suffering, towards or from another, during sexual behaviour. These disorders may be encountered in association with, or secondary to, another psychiatric disorder. Sometimes the individuals themselves present if the behaviour is perceived as wrong or distressing, or they may be referred for assessment following a sexual offence.

Fetishism

A person with fetishism desires, and is sexually gratified by non-living objects such as specific articles of clothing. Without these objects, sexual dysfunction usually results.

Fetishistic transvestism

In fetishistic transvestism, clothing of the opposite sex is worn (cross-dressing) to achieve sexual excitement, usually by masturbation. This can vary in extent from one or two articles worn for short periods, to complete and permanent cross-dressing.

Exhibitionism

The individual with exhibitionism has strong sexually arousing fantasies of, and sexual urges for, exposing their genitals to others. The act itself is usually accompanied by sexual arousal and may involve masturbation.

General medical causes of sexual dysfunction	
System	**Disorder**
endocrine	diabetes mellitus hypothyroidism hyper/hypoadrenocorticism hyperprolactinaemia
neurological	multiple sclerosis peripheral neuropathy spinal cord injury
reproductive	pelvic surgery or irradiation atrophic vaginitis endometriosis pelvic infection
other	peripheral vascular disease renal failure debilitating disease, e.g. COAD physical disability/deformity

Fig. 10.2 General medical causes of sexual dysfunction.

Prescribed drug and illicit substance causes of sexual dysfunction	
alcohol amphetamine anabolic steroids anticonvulsants antidepressants antihistamines antihypertensives	antipsychotics benzodiazepines cocaine contraceptive pill diuretics opioids

Fig. 10.3 Prescribed drug and illicit substance causes of sexual dysfunction.

Voyeurism

In voyeurism, sexual fantasies and arousal are associated with watching the sexual behaviour of others or watching others undress. Again, this is often accompanied by masturbation.

Paedophilia

Paedophilia refers to a disorder in which early pubertal or prepubertal children form the focus of sexual fantasies and activity (although some individuals in adult relationships retain the fantasies only).

Sadomasochism

Sadomasochism involves fantasies of, and urges for, participating in sexual activity which involves the infliction of pain or humiliation, such as beating and bondage. An individual may prefer to be the inflictor or the recipient. The diagnosis requires caution as infliction of pain and suffering is commonly incorporated into sexual activity to enhance enjoyment and arousal. As with all other paraphilias, sadomasochism must be the primary focus of sexual excitement.

Other paraphilias

Other disorders of sexual preference include:
- Zoophilia (animals).
- Necrophilia (corpses).
- Telephone scatologia (obscene telephone calls).
- Frotteurism (touching and rubbing against a non-consenting person).

Differential diagnosis

Like personality disorders, the paraphilias can usually be traced to a person's early psychosexual development (i.e. in childhood and adolescence). Inappropriate sexual behaviour is commonly associated with learning disability. When there is a more rapid change in sexual fantasies and behaviour, particularly in middle or old age, it is important to exclude an underlying disorder which may be affecting beliefs, judgement, sexual drive, and impulse control. Always consider dementia, organic personality change, psychotic disorders, and severe mood disorders in these circumstances.

Gender identity disorders

Persons with gender identity disorders are uncomfortable with their own anatomical sex, and attempt to adopt the appearance and characteristics of the opposite gender.

Transsexualism

Transsexualism manifests in adulthood and is characterized by:
- A preoccupation with having been born the wrong sex.
- Cross-dressing.
- Adopting the mannerisms and behaviour of the opposite sex.
- Attempts to minimize or remove one's primary and secondary sexual characteristics.

Psychiatrists may be asked to assess these patients prior to sex hormone or surgical treatment. In addition, the personal and social consequences of transsexualism, such as rejection by family and stigmatization, frequently lead to mood and substance-use disorders. These patients have an increased risk of suicide and self-harm.

Differential diagnosis

Transsexualism must be distinguished from fetishistic transvestism: in the former, cross-dressing arises secondary to the person's belief that they are the wrong gender; whereas in the latter, cross-dressing facilitates sexual excitement and pleasure (a minority do eventually develop a gender identity disorder).

The other main differential, a psychotic disorder, arises when the belief of being the wrong biological sex or gender is delusional. Transsexuals accept they were born a specific biological sex but feel they are the wrong gender.

Eliciting psychosexual histories is one of the more neglected areas of history-taking, often because of the interviewer's fear and embarrassment. Enquiry requires sensitivity and tact; it is best to question this area in detail after sufficient rapport has been made, perhaps at the end of the history. Sexual abuse, although a particularly sensitive area, is an important risk factor for future psychiatric disorder (and is often not reported in histories). An opening question might be: 'I realize this may be a difficult area, but we ask this question of everyone as we hear of it so much nowadays . . . Were you ever harmed or abused in the past?'. Always remember not to pursue the details if the patient is unwilling to talk about it, and never put words in their mouth.

11. Childhood Problems

Mrs CD brings her 10-year-old son to the child psychiatry clinic. The family were referred at the request of the school, who had noticed increasing problems with his behaviour. This took the form of aggressive outbursts directed towards both staff and other pupils, and difficulty keeping up with his school-work through poor attention and overactivity. Mrs CD said he behaved similarly at home, appearing to deteriorate following her separation from Mr CD. She added that he had started to soil his underpants and wet his bed at night.

Psychopathology

Most medical students gain a little experience of child and adolescent psychiatry in clinical attachments. It is a large specialty within psychiatry and has important differences to adult psychiatry, both in the approach to assessment and treatment and in the disorders encountered. This chapter and the corresponding chapter in Part III (see Chapter 24) are designed to give an introduction to this area.

When considering the problems presenting to child psychiatry, these points need to be borne in mind:

- Problems need to be seen in the context of a child's developmental stage; for example, temper tantrums are normal at 2 years but should start to subside by 5 years.
- The 'problem' is usually presented by someone else, e.g. parent, paediatrician, school. It is often presented in terms of abnormal behaviour (e.g. school refusal) rather than psychological symptoms.

Disorders recognized in childhood can generally be classified in terms of:

- Abnormal psychological development.
- Acquired disorders specific to childhood.
- 'Adult' disorders developing or occurring in childhood.

These can be summarized in a diagnostic algorithm (Fig. 11.1).

Differential diagnosis
Mental retardation

In the United Kingdom, the less pejorative term 'learning disability' is used in preference to 'mental retardation'. It denotes a global impairment of learning skills which emerges during development and persists through adult life.

Learning disabilities are normally detected when a child demonstrates a delay in acquiring appropriate cognitive, language, social, and motor skills for his or her age. Consequently, measures of overall intelligence are below population norms, where an IQ of less than 70 is regarded as the cut-off point. The more severe the disability, the earlier a delay is recognized.

The four grades of learning disability are shown in Fig. 11.2

Learning disability may coexist with another developmental disorder (e.g. autism) or with a physical illness or disability (e.g. epilepsy). There is also an increased risk of developing another psychiatric disorder (e.g. schizophrenia), and these are particularly important to exclude whenever there is any change in emotions or behaviour from previous patterns.

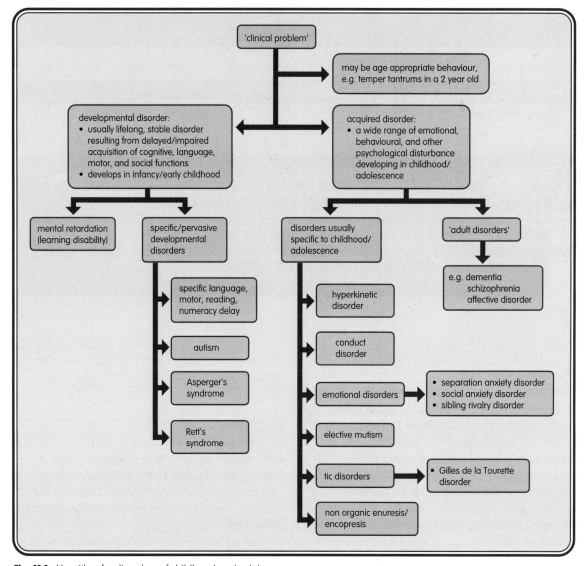

Fig. 11.1 Algorithm for disorders of childhood and adolescence.

Specific developmental disorder

Specific developmental disorders closely resemble the previous category in that they describe impaired or delayed development arising in early life which is usually stable through adult life.

The disorders may be:

- Of specific function (e.g. language, reading, numeracy, or motor skills).
- Pervasive development disorders.

Specific function disorders

In specific function disorders, the impairment occurs in the absence of a global learning difficulty, so that other areas of function are average or above. Compared with learning disability, the person has less difficulty with overall social and personal functioning, although the consequences of a delay, for example with reading skills ('dyslexia'), may result in other emotional or behavioural problems.

Fig. 11.2 Grades of learning disability.

Grades of learning disability		
Grade of disability	**IQ (mental age)**	**Functioning**
mild	50–69 (8–12 years)	usually acquire language and independent living skills but significant academic difficulties (e.g. reading/writing) and social immaturity (e.g. occupational, child-rearing difficulties)
moderate	35–49 (3–8 years)	only minority able to live independently and ~50% have severe language difficulties; minority develop literacy
severe	20–34 (1–3 years)	majority do not develop speech, often a physical disability, require life-long care
profound	<20 (<1 year)	limited language skills (basic audio/visual commands), usually severe physical disability, require nursing care

Pervasive development disorders

Autism This disorder emerges in the first 3 years of life and is characterized by:

- Abnormal social interaction—e.g. failure to initiate, develop, or respond to social interaction; poor grasp of non-verbal social cues, avoidance of eye-to-eye contact.
- Impaired communication skills—e.g. delayed or impaired language development, difficulty maintaining conversation, lack of creativity or age-appropriate play.
- Restricted and repetitive behaviour—e.g. rigid and routine interests and activities, preoccupation with dates or numbers, motor stereotypies (see Chapter 13).

Approximately 75% of autistic children have a learning disability. Other problems associated with this disorder are phobias, aggression, self-injury, sleep and eating disorders, and epilepsy.

Asperger's syndrome This is thought to be closely related to autism and shares the core symptoms of impaired social interaction and restricted, stereotyped behaviour (e.g. preoccupation with bus timetables). However, individuals do not have a learning difficulty and usually lead independent, successful lives. As intelligence is normal, it usually presents later than

autism, often at school through social awkwardness and motor clumsiness. In adult life individuals may be considered as eccentric or odd, and may resemble those with schizoid or anankastic personality disorders.

Rett's syndrome This is a disorder specific to girls and is characterized by the development of severe learning disability during the first 2 years of life. After initial normal development, language skills become impaired and fine motor skills are lost, commonly being replaced by stereotypical 'hand wringing'. There is deceleration of head growth, excess salivation, tongue protrusion, scoliosis, and loss of sphincter control. Epilepsy, ataxia, and spinal atrophy often occur.

Disorders specific to childhood
Hyperkinetic disorder (attention deficit hyperactivity disorder—ADHD)

There are three core features of hyperkinetic disorder:

- Inattention—the child is easily distractible, forgetful, avoids tasks requiring concentration, and has difficulty sustaining play and academic tasks.
- Overactivity—the child is fidgety, reckless, socially disinhibited, talks excessively, and is inappropriately active.
- Impulsivity—the child persistently interrupts and intrudes; they are unable to wait their turn.

The disorder is not usually recognized until the child has started school, although very severe cases may present in preschool children. To help differentiate from normal childhood behaviour, it must be shown to interfere with the child's social and academic progress. The disorder is more common among learning-disabled children and there is often overlap with conduct disorder (see below).

Conduct disorder

The core features of conduct disorder are a persistent pattern of:

- Increased aggression towards other people or animals.
- Violation of rules and regulations, e.g. theft, property damage, truancy.
- Deceitfulness, frequently associated with loss of empathy towards others.

Beneath an aggressive and defiant exterior, there is usually low self-esteem, and this group are at an increased risk of attempted suicide. Their behaviour may lead to school expulsion, juvenile crime, and institutional care. Other behaviours include substance misuse, promiscuity, and prostitution.

It is a chronic disorder and usually presents in late childhood or adolescence.

Conduct disorder should not be used to label isolated acts of delinquency or behaviour that is culturally acceptable to the child but unacceptable to the observer.

Associated disorders include learning disability (both global and specific), hyperkinetic disorder, and emotional disorder (see below).

Emotional disorders

Along with conduct disorder, emotional disorders are the most common presentations to child psychiatry. They encompass the depressive, stress-related, and anxiety disorders discussed elsewhere and several distinct disorders of childhood listed below:

- Separation anxiety disorder— excessive anxiety over separation (real or imagined) from a parent or other important figure; this leads to preoccupying worry over separation and often manifests as refusal to attend school.
- Social anxiety disorder—excessive fear of strangers beyond that which normally develops in the first year of life.
- Sibling rivalry disorder—although a degree of emotional disturbance occurs in most children after a sibling is born, sometimes the behavioural manifestations are particularly persistent and severe, with marked hostility and aggression.

Elective mutism

Elective mutism usually develops in early childhood and presents as an apparent inability to speak in certain situations. Prior language development is usually normal, although a minority of cases have a pre-existing global or specific learning disability. It often occurs as a consequence of a severe psychosocial stress such as bereavement.

Tic disorders

A tic is a sudden, repetitive movement varying in complexity from eye blinking and arm jerking to jumping and facial gestures. Vocal tics may range from simple snorts or barks to complex words.

The sufferer has some degree of voluntary control over the movements and they diminish in sleep. This differs from the involuntary movements of other movement disorders such as Huntington's disease (see Chapter 6) or tardive dyskinesia (see Chapter 15). Another important differential are the more purposeful motor stereotypies and mannerisms seen in autism and catatonia (see Chapter 15).

Gilles de la Tourette disorder is a disabling condition characterized by both motor and vocal tics. The obscene vocal tics, or coprolalia, classically associated with this disorder are only present in a minority.

Non-organic enuresis and non-organic encopresis

Non-organic enuresis and non-organic encopresis refer to the voluntary or involuntary voiding of urine and faeces, respectively, in an inappropriate location when an organic cause (e.g. urinary tract infection or laxative abuse) is absent. Because both occur normally in early development, enuresis is not normally diagnosed until 5 years and encopresis until 4 years. Nocturnal enuresis (bed wetting), in particular, may persist until late adolescence. Either disorder may reflect an underlying psychological stress or present as part of an emotional disorder. The behaviour itself can lead to distress through embarrassment and ostracism.

Adult disorders in childhood

Psychiatric disorders encountered in adults may occur during childhood and specific features relating to the presentation of the most significant of these are shown in Fig. 11.3.

Discussion of vignette
What is the boy's differential diagnosis?

The presentation has elements of several disorders:

- Conduct disorder—aggression and bullying.
- Hyperkinetic disorder—inattention and overactivity.
- Global or specific learning difficulty—falling behind at school.
- Emotional disorder, e.g. depression—tearfulness and irritability.
- Nocturnal enuresis and encopresis.

Of significance in the history is his parents' recent separation, which may have been extremely traumatic for the child. The behaviours could be explained by an adjustment disorder.

What further information could clarify the diagnosis?

The important question is how far the boy's difficulties predate the apparent stress of parental

Adult psychiatric disorders in childhood	
Disorder	**Comments**
dementia/delirium	dementia extremely rare, e.g. CJD, SSPE, Huntington's disease, HIV delirium common during febrile illnesses young children
substance misuse disorders	predominantly alcohol, cannabis and inhalants during adolescence
schizophrenia	extremely rare before 7 years, increasing incidence in adolescence, male>female. Tend to present with thought disorder and blunted/inappropriate affect, rather than frank delusions or hallucinations
bipolar disorder	up to 25% of cases first present in adolescence although very rare before puberty
depressive disorders	children and young adolescents are less sophisticated in their expression of feelings; cognitive and somatic symptoms of depression are less readily identified. Depression often presents with tearfulness, anhedonia, irritability, and non-specific somatic symptoms. Anxiety, conduct and eating disorders are commonly associated
anxiety disorders	less likely to present with typical somatic or depersonalization/derealization symptoms of anxiety. May present with school refusal, social withdrawal, non-specific physical complaints, enuresis or encopresis. Specific phobias are common in this age group
obsessive–compulsive disorder	children often develop mild obsessions, magical thinking and rituals; occasionally true OCD develops
suicide	rare in this age group (1 per million 10–14years/year, 50 per million 15–19years/year) rate appears to be increasing among adolescents. Male>female; associated with conduct disorder, depressive disorder, child abuse, and family history of suicide
CJD=Creutzfeld-Jacob disease, SSPE= Subacute sclerosing pan-encephalitis	

Fig. 11.3 Adult psychiatric disorders in childhood.

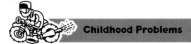

separation. His 'problem' may have been indirectly exaggerated by factors at school (e.g. reorganization, new teacher) or at home (e.g. financial insecurity, mother adapting to stresses of being a lone parent). Therefore, assessment should carefully consider the following:

- Developmental history—pregnancy and birth complications, attainment of developmental milestones, childhood illnesses, preschool personality.
- School history—problems with attendance and behaviour, academic abilities (this could be clarified by a report from an educational psychologist), social skills.
- Family history—this should be elaborated to include enquiry into family relationships, reaction to previous losses and separation, physical and psychiatric illness within the family, and quality of early environment.
- Current problems—in this age group, other problems that might clarify the diagnosis include school refusal, physical symptoms, anxiety symptoms, sleep and eating disturbances, and ritualistic or obsessional behaviour.

What are the general principles of assessment in child and adolescent psychiatry?

Unlike in adult psychiatry where the majority of patients self present, children and adolescents almost always accompany carers.

Children and young adolescents are usually first interviewed with carers, who predominantly define the symptoms. Nevertheless, the child's feelings and understanding of the problem can be assessed, either directly by questioning or indirectly by observing their behaviour and play during the session. This also gives an insight into their cognitive and physical development as well as patterns of family interaction.

Older adolescents are more capable of expressing their feelings in an adult fashion and it is useful to interview them alone as well as with carers. Rapport is often difficult to attain initially as interviewers may be viewed with suspicion, as an authority figure or as siding with carers. It is important to maintain neutrality and not appear to side with either adolescent or carer.

When children under 16 are considered to be mature enough to give valid consent, their rights to confidentiality and consent to treatment should be upheld; always seek legal advice if you are unsure.

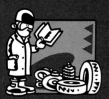

12. Suicide Attempt

THE PATIENT WHO HAS ATTEMPTED SUICIDE

At 1.30 a.m. the psychiatry senior house officer receives a call from the casualty department in the main city teaching hospital. He is asked to assess a 24-year-old unemployed single man, Mr SA, who was brought in by his landlord. The landlord had called round on the off chance to discuss payment arrears, only to find the door unlocked and Mr SA asleep on his bed with a large but empty bottle of paracetamol tablets and several empty cans of lager littered around the bedroom floor. Mr SA was easily roused but was abusive to the landlord's persistent pleas that they should go along to the hospital. Only when he was violently sick did he finally agree. The casualty officer reports that the patient has had a thorough medical examination and investigations. Paracetamol was detected in his blood but not at a sufficiently high level to require medical admission. He is now considerably calmer but refutes any attempt to talk about what happened—he insists that he just wants to go home.

Psychopathology
Suicide
Suicide is the act of intentionally bring about one's own death. Suicide may be achieved by self-poisoning (by drugs or poisonous substances such as carbon monoxide) or by more violent means (e.g. jumping from heights, hanging, or use of firearms).

Parasuicide
Parasuicide refers to any act that mimics suicide but does not result in death. The patient knowingly ingests an excess of a substance that they believe to be active or poisonous, or engages in an activity such as jumping from a height, but survives.

Individuals who engage in parasuicidal acts vary widely in their actual intent. A proportion fully intend to kill themselves but are thwarted either by chance discovery by a friend or relative or by misjudgement in their method of attempted suicide, such as taking too few tablets or having effective intake minimized by vomiting.

When performing a mental state examination you should always ask the patient whether they have had thoughts of deliberately ending their own life and whether they are still having any such thoughts. Suicidal ideation varies, from occasional fleeting suicidal thoughts which are soon dismissed when life's challenges or responsibilities are considered, to elaborate plans with the location, method, and associated issues like a 'final act' or the leaving of a note all carefully considered.

Some will later report that their attempt was founded on a sudden impulsive wish to escape from life's stresses and that they made a 'spur of the moment' decision to try and bring about this escape. Others describe a behaviour motivated by the desire to make those around them take more notice of their problems—a so-called 'cry-for-help' parasuicide—or even to make others feel guilty.

Although these categories may appear clear-cut, it must be remembered that because over half of those engaging in parasuicidal behaviour do so when under the influence of alcohol, it is often difficult to tease out the true motive of the attempt.

Deliberate self-harm

Deliberate self-harm refers to any intentionally self-inflicted damage to one's own body, irrespective of whether it is minor or potentially life-threatening. Actions from superficial cuts in the forearm to serious parasuicides are included.

Assessing risk of suicide

Epidemiological risk factors

Risk factors for both parasuicide and completed suicide include:

- Having performed one or more parasuicidal acts.
- Being single, separated, or divorced.
- Having a lack of employment (including the retired).
- Living alone and being socially isolated.

Males are more likely to complete suicide than females, although females engage in more parasuicidal acts. Elderly males have the highest suicide risk with a smaller peak in males aged 16–25 years. A family history of depression and suicide also increase the risk of completed suicide.

Physical illness

Any disabling or unpleasant medical condition may be related to suicide. Examples include:

- Central nervous system diseases, e.g. epilepsy, multiple sclerosis, Huntington's disease.
- Cancers, especially of the genitals or breast.
- Endocrine conditions, e.g. Cushing's disease.
- Metabolic abnormalities, e.g. porphyria.

Psychiatric illness

Ninety-five percent of those who take their own life and the majority of those who perform parasuicidal acts have a psychiatric disorder.

Depressive disorders are the most common. Look closely for anhedonia and cognitive symptoms such as feelings of hopelessness and worthlessness. The risk is greatest when depression is associated with delusions.

Alcohol dependence is associated with a 15-fold increase in suicide risk, and dependence on heroin with a 20-fold increase, compared with the general population. Alcohol and substance abuse are also associated with an increased parasuicide rate. Most of the alcoholics who commit suicide also have a depressive disorder, and alcohol dependence is itself correlated with risk factors for suicide such as lack of employment and social isolation.

Schizophrenia is also associated with higher suicide rates than the general population. Some schizophrenic patients attempt suicide in response to threatening voices inciting self-harm (command hallucinations), or as a consequence of delusions of persecution or control by an external force bent on making the patient harm themself. Episodes of illness may be associated with poor control of impulses, feelings of emptiness, and the need to escape from the recurrent gross mental disturbance. Young male patients with good educational records and high ambitions prior to development of schizophrenia are at high risk, as are those who live alone or are dependent on psychiatric services.

Certain personality disorders such as borderline and dissocial have an association with parasuicide. Borderline patients who are uncertain of their own image, make poor relationships but beg to avoid rejection, and may feel alone and empty, are particularly prone to repeated acts of deliberate self-harm.

Anxiety disorder such as panic disorder, and eating disorders such as anorexia, are also thought to be associated with an increased risk of suicidal activity.

Other predisposing, provoking, and perpetuating factors

The psychiatric history should as usual include an assessment of all of the patient's current problems in life, considering home circumstances, relationships, and other factors which may predispose to suicidal ideation or activity, provoke an attempt, or perpetuate suicidal thoughts.

Assessment of the patient who has attempted suicide

Around 25% of parasuicidal acts are followed by another within a year. The level of risk of further parasuicide or completed suicide must be assessed.

A thorough risk assessment should include:
- A full psychiatric history with specific enquiry about the dynamics of and method used for the suicide attempt (with the likelihood of its success or of being discovered before any real damage is done), the motive or intent, and the presence of the epidemiological, physical, psychiatric, and other risk factors outlined above.
- A mental state examination.
- An assessment of the patient's current situation with emphasis on any circumstance that has altered since the attempt.

Method
Suicide attempts are most commonly through:
- Self-poisoning—by tablet overdoses, ingestion of poison, or inhalation of carbon monoxide gas from car exhausts.
- More violent means—jumping from heights, use of firearms, hanging, or electrocution.

An assessment should be made as to the likelihood of the method used causing death. Although deaths have been reported after ingestion of less than 5 g of paracetamol, such an action is much less likely to be fatal than a plunge from a tenth-floor balcony. However, use of an apparently ineffective method (e.g. taking six paracetamol tablets) may reflect lack of knowledge of the dose needed rather than a lack of intent to die. Further questions about the method which may be helpful in assessing the motive for the attempt are:
- How much forward planning went into the attempt? A serious attempt may involve complex and meticulous planning, including perhaps a suicide note, or performance of a 'final act'.
- What was the likelihood of discovery or rescue? Contrast the lonesome Mr SA, who was only discovered by a chance visit from a landlord, to the young lady who takes a mouthful of tablets and then runs downstairs to her parents to reveal what she has done.

Motive
Did the patient genuinely wish to end their life and did they expect to live or to die from the means they used in the attempt?

Some patients are quite open about their motive: they may express a continued wish to die and regret that their attempt failed; alternatively, they may admit to making a

Parasuicide may reflect:
- A long-established wish to die which might have been carried through but for chance discovery or failure to absorb sufficient of a toxic substance.
- A spur of the moment decision to escape from life's problems.
- A wish to alert others to their problems and effect change rather than a wish to to die.

cry for help and may now be quite embarrassed. Others are less co-operative and it may take some time before their true intent can be established.

Mental state
Define the patient's mental state by checking:
- What is their mood at present and is it associated with features such as hopelessness, worthlessness, and guilt, or with anger or rage?
- Is continuing suicidal ideation expressed and if not could a strong wish to die be being concealed?
- Is there any evidence of psychotic features? For instance, a schizophrenic patient may attempt suicide in response to command hallucinations or through delusions of control.

Assessment of current situation
Assess the current situation by checking:
- Has there been any change in the individual's circumstances since the parasuicidal act was committed? The action may have evoked sympathy and made carers and associates wish to give more time and attention to the patient, but, of course, the opposite may have happened.
- What is the level of social support?
- Does the individual have the resources and ability to cope if discharged?

Discussion of vignette
Mr SA's reluctance to talk to the on-call psychiatrist makes an assessment of risk difficult. If he cannot give

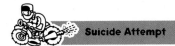

a proper history, information from the landlord and from any available neighbour, friend, or relative will be of value.

What epidemiological risk factors for suicidal activity does Mr SA carry?

As well as being a 24 year old male, Mr SA is single, lives alone in apparent social isolation, and is unemployed.

Is there any evidence of psychiatric illness?

The landlord's report of lager cans strewn around the floor raises the suspicion that Mr SA may be suffering from an alcohol problem, although it is possible that he has merely engaged in a one-off alcohol binge. Given the substantial suicide risk among alcoholics, it would be necessary to investigate this possibility thoroughly (see Chapter 7). He also carries a risk of depression through the risk factors discussed above, so enquiries should be made regarding depressive symptoms.

Have predisposing, provoking, or perpetuating factors emerged?

There is some suggestion of acute financial trouble which could have provoked the attempt. Further factors may become apparent—for example, news

of his suicide attempt may filter through to an estranged partner whose attitude to Mr SA may become more sympathetic, improving his prospects on discharge.

From the landlord's information what inferences can we make about method and motive?

It appears that Mr SA attempted to consume enough paracetamol tablets to cause real harm, and the fact that he would not have been discovered but for the landlord's timely arrival points towards a degree of forward planning. There may be some ambivalence as he left the door unlocked and was willing to go to hospital after vomiting.

What would the on-call psychiatrist do next?

The many unanswered questions, the apparent lack of home support, and the difficulty in completing an assessment that has already shown the presence of several risk factors make it likely that Mr SA would be admitted to an inpatient unit. His mental state and in particular on-going suicidal ideation could be properly examined, the gaps in the history filled in and the presence of depression or other psychiatric disorders assessed.

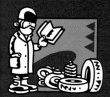

THE PSYCHIATRIC PATIENT WHO DOES NOT COMMUNICATE

A medical student nearing the psychiatry exam picks a patient—Mr NC, aged 54—at random from the list of inpatients on an acute general adult psychiatry ward. She enters Mr NC's room and introduces herself: he does not reply. She asks a question: again there is no response. For a moment the medical student wonders whether Mr NC is actually conscious, but she decides that he must be as his eyes are following her vigilantly as she moves around the room. There are no other signs of voluntary movement except that every few seconds Mr NC raises his right hand and makes a gesture resembling a salute. The student grasps Mr NC's hand and notes that muscle tone is normal, but when there is still no response she comes to the conclusion that verbal interaction will not be possible and leaves to discuss the patient with the ward staff.

Psychopathology

Negative symptoms of schizophrenia

Positive symptoms of schizophrenia such as delusions and hallucinations have been described in Chapter 5. When schizophrenia is chronic, negative symptoms may predominate. These include:

- Flattening or blunting of affect—manifest by failure to show signs of expressing emotion, e.g. monotonous voice, lack of facial expression.
- Poverty of speech—verbal responses become vague or involve a limited range of phrases.
- Lack of motivation.
- Anhedonia (see Chapter 1).

Negative symptoms have traditionally been difficult to treat by conventional neuroleptic drugs and have tended to be long-lasting. However, the newer, atypical antipsychotic drugs have been shown to be effective against these symptoms. This may help to reduce the progressive deterioration in social functioning seen currently in many chronic schizophrenics with uncontrolled negative symptoms.

Stupor

In stupor, a patient remains conscious but appears to be unaware of their surroundings and makes no or little spontaneous movement except for their eyes. The patient can sometimes recall the stuporous period when it has passed.

Catatonic symptoms

Catatonic features may be associated with schizophrenia or with severe depressive episodes but are now rare in western societies. They include:

- Motoric immobility—catalepsy, waxy flexibility, and catatonic stupor. Catalepsy refers to the maintenance of an immobile position for long

Stupor can be precipitated by dissociative disorders (see Chapter 4), as well as by catatonic schizophrenia, manic episodes, severe depression, or organic factors. For dissociative stupor to be diagnosed, it is necessary to establish that a patient has been subject to recent stress-provoking events.

periods. In waxy flexibility, muscle tone is such that the patient's limbs may be moved slowly to any position the examiner desires; the new position, however bizarre, is then maintained for some time.

- Automatic obedience—instructions, whether sensible or pointless, are carried out in a robot-like fashion.
- Negativism—the patient resists all instructions with no apparent motive and maintains a rigid posture against attempts to be moved.
- Mutism.
- Posturing—bizarre positions are voluntarily assumed.
- Mannerisms—apparently goal-directed movements (e.g. waving, saluting) which are repeated frequently and inappropriately.
- Stereotypies—fixed pattern of movements (e.g. rocking, gyrating) which occur frequently and lack the apparent significance of mannerisms.
- Echopraxia—imitation of the interviewer's movements and posture.
- Echolalia—inappropriate repetition of the interviewer's words.

Differential diagnosis

There are various possible explanations as to why a patient might make no verbal communication and display such limited voluntary movements in the presence of an interviewer. These include:

- A deliberate decision to say nothing and sit still as they do not wish to help by discussing their case (this explanation may apply to an angry or grandiose patient).
- A deliberate decision to say nothing and sit still as this might be reported back and add to the perceived seriousness of the case (e.g. malingering) or because of a desire to produce such symptoms without an obvious motivation (factitious disorder).
- The existence of a chronic general medical condition (e.g. motor neuron disease, old cerebrovascular accident) or an acute medical problem (e.g. head injury, acute cerebrovascular accident) which prevents them from responding. This may give rise to organic stupor, or be a manifestation of a larger picture of delirium or dementia (see Chapter 5).
- The influence of a prescribed drug (e.g. an antipsychotic) or an illicit substance which prevents a response. Neuroleptic malignant syndrome, a movement disorder caused by

antipsychotics, is a dangerous condition in which muscular rigidity and dystonia are accompanied by mutism, agitation, fever, and increased blood pressure (see Chapter 15).

- A lack of motivation to respond caused by severe depression with marked psychomotor retardation or by schizophrenia with negative symptoms.
- A period of stupor secondary to severe depression, to a pronounced manic episode, to schizophrenia with catatonic features, organic factors, or to a recent stressful event (dissociative stupor).

Discussion of vignette

Some patients are either unwilling or unable to communicate, or communicate very sparingly.

Although the medical student was unable to take a history from Mr NC, his case can still provide an educational insight. A discussion with the ward staff and with relatives or carers would be useful—when a psychiatrist meets an uncommunicative patient for the first time, such liaison is essential.

What possible diagnoses need to be ruled out quickly?

The medical student should establish whether Mr NC's lack of communication represents a sudden change from his normal state: if it does, it would be necessary to alert a clinician to rule out the acute onset of a medical problem such as a head injury or new cerebral infarct. A substance-related cause should also be considered (see Chapter 7): the patient may have ingested an illicit substance or may have neuroleptic malignant syndrome.

Assuming Mr NC is known to have a chronic psychiatric illness, can you spot an additional feature that points to a likely diagnosis?

If Mr NC was known to already have features of depression or chronic schizophrenia, it is likely that his behaviour represents a continuation of these illnesses. He may be exhibiting a gross lack of motivation to move and communicate. Mutism, immobility, and stupor could be associated with appearance of the catatonic features of either schizophrenia or severe depression, and Mr NC is exhibiting one further sign which is suggestive of this: the recurrent raising of his hand to make a movement that resembles a salute is likely to be a mannerism, another sign of catatonia.

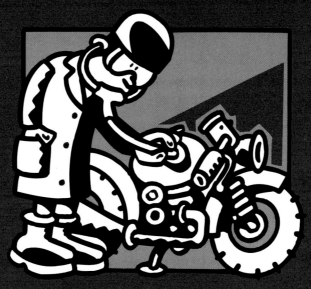

HISTORY, EXAMINATION, AND COMMON INVESTIGATIONS

14. Assessing Patients

AIMS OF THE HISTORY AND MENTAL STATE EXAMINATION

When a clinician takes a psychiatric history and performs a mental state examination, the main aims are:
- To gain information which may help the interviewer to understand the patient's problems and their impact on the patient's life.
- To obtain sufficient details to make a formulation of possible diagnoses and draw up a management plan.
- To improve the relationship between the clinician and the patient.

For medical students and clinicians seeking to sharpen their skills, history taking and mental state examination also serve as one of the best ways of improving techniques and broadening knowledge of psychiatric conditions by talking with patients first-hand.

When introducing yourself to a patient:
- Be confident—but don't be arrogant!
- Describing yourself as a 'student doctor' tends to cut more ice with patients than using the term 'medical student'.
- Asking a ward doctor or nurse to introduce you can be helpful.
- It is sensible to mention the name of the consultant to whom you are attached and explain that you have some specific questions to ask as part of your training.

INTERVIEW TECHNIQUE

The interview must be conducted in a setting where both parties feel safe and privacy can be respected. It is important to establish rapport with the patient, identifying yourself and explaining why you wish to conduct the interview—especially as some psychiatric patients may be suspicious of 'outsiders' or reluctant to co-operate with those who are allied to the medical profession.

Exams are a little different in that the patients are expecting to be interviewed and examined by the candidates. Some may be seasoned campaigners who are brought in especially—they are generally keen to help and are well aware of the format. Other 'volunteers' may be recruited from the wards—they may be less enthusiastic or may not have realized the time-pressures that the candidates are under.

When taking a psychiatric history and performing a mental state examination you will need to:

- Be systematic in obtaining the necessary information.
- Ask open and closed questions (see 'Presenting complaint' section).
- Listen to the answers and use the information to formulate further relevant questions.
- Be empathic and show understanding in comments you make, and, if necessary, tailor your questions to the patient.
- Redirect the conversation if the patient has taken the interview away from relevant issues.
- Pick up non-verbal information from the patient's appearance and behaviour, and make further objective assessments (e.g. mood, speech) for the mental state examination.
- Make notes during the interview if possible (essential in an exam).

It may also be appropriate to take a history from a relative or carer, especially in the situations listed in Fig. 14.1.

Examples of problems where a corroborative history is useful	
Problem	**Reason for needing collaborative history**
cognitive impairment lack of insight active psychotic illness severe learning disability	patient unable to understand or to respond to questions appropriately
alcohol/drug problems suicide attempts	patient's responses may be unreliable or misleading
sleep problems	difficult to assess quantity and quality of one's own sleep

Fig. 14.1 Examples of problems where a corroborative history is useful.

CONTENTS OF THE PSYCHIATRIC HISTORY

The psychiatric history can be divided into three sections:
- Introductory information.
- Presenting complaint(s) and history of presenting complaint(s).
- Other psychiatric, medical, and personal history.

Introductory information
The following details should be obtained at the start of the history:
- Patient's name.
- Patient's age.
- Patient's occupation.
- The reason for the patient's presence in the psychiatric setting (e.g. referral to outpatients by family doctor, admitted to ward informally having presented at casualty).
- Mental Health Act status if detained under a section (see Chapter 16).

In practice, this information is often available before the patient is actually seen, and can be used for presentation as a concise opening statement: 'Mr Roger Brown is a 62-year-old retired schoolteacher who was referred to outpatients by his family doctor . . . '.

Presenting complaint(s) and history of presenting complaint(s)
The 'battle' of taking, organizing, and presenting a psychiatric history is usually won and lost here.

As in any medical history, open questions (e.g. 'What are your problems?' or 'What's brought you to see a psychiatrist?') are better than closed questions (e.g. 'Do you have depression?') at the beginning to allow the patient to identify problems without being affected by the interviewer's agenda. It is then appropriate to move progressively to more closed questions to obtain specific details.

Presenting complaint(s)
The presenting complaint consists of a list of one or more distinct problems of which the patient complains—using their own words if possible rather than altering them to stricter medical terminology, e.g.:
- He complains of 'feeling down all the time'.
- He complains firstly of being 'depressed', secondly of having 'occasional highs', and thirdly of having alcohol problems.

History of presenting complaint(s)
The history of the presenting complaint involves thorough questioning about each of the distinct problems listed under 'presenting complaint'.

The nature of each presenting problem can be described under the following headings:
- Time.
- Course.
- Progression.
- Associated symptoms.
- Severity.
- Predisposing, precipitating, and perpetuating factors.

It is helpful to organize multiple presenting complaints into groups of symptoms which constitute 'distinct problems'. When a patient presents with many symptoms, group together those which are likely to be part of the same disease: for example, 'feeling sad', 'lacking motivation', and 'having no energy' are all common features of depressive episodes and can subsequently be described together as one presenting complaint. However, if a quite different symptom is also present (e.g. deliberate vomiting of food), present its onset, course, and development as a separate distinct problem.

Time

Check:

- When was the problem first noticed?

Course

Since its onset, has the problem been:

- Constant?
- Progressively getting worse?
- Intermittent or recurrent—with partial or complete recovery between episodes?

If a distinct episode of the present problem has occurred before, it is normally better to concentrate on the present episode, leaving the earlier ones to the past psychiatric history. However, there may be instances where the distinction between episodes is blurred, or a fluctuating symptom has become intolerable because it has been long-lasting—in cases such as these, all of the details can be included in history of presenting complaint.

Progression

Does the problem consist of:

- One symptom only?

- One symptom initially, with subsequent development of associated symptoms (see below).
- Multiple symptoms from the onset?

Associated symptoms

When the presenting complaint is a problem that is a feature of one or more of the psychiatric illnesses described in this book, time should be taken to explore whether any other symptoms that typically occur in those illnesses are present.

For example, mention of 'feeling low' as a presenting complaint should trigger questions about biological, cognitive, and somatic features of depression—the object being to see whether there are sufficient symptoms for depressive disorder to be a likely diagnosis.

As discussed in Chapter 1, low mood may exist in other psychiatric illnesses such as bipolar affective disorder, so further questions need to be asked about symptoms of these disorders (e.g. 'Have you experienced periods of feeling inordinately happy or elated?'). As depression often involves psychotic features, questions on delusions and hallucinations should also be asked.

Rather than immediately complaining of 'feeling low' a patient might cite 'poor concentration' and 'lack of motivation' as their main problems. Both may be symptoms of depression, so this possibility should be explored with questions on low mood and other depressive symptoms. They can also occur in schizophrenia and delusional disorders, so questions on these illnesses are, again, relevant.

Severity

Find out:

- Are the patient's symptoms severe and distressing or are they mild?
- To what extent do they interfere with the patient's life (e.g. employment, education, and relationships)?

Predisposing, precipitating, and perpetuating factors

Find out:

- Is the patient aware of any traits, events, or other factors that were evident before the problem appeared which might have made them vulnerable to developing it?
- Did any event or action occur just before the onset of the problem or coincide with it? Does any factor

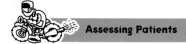

appear to regularly provoke onset of symptoms or make the symptoms worse?

- Is there any factor that appears to prevent the patient from finding relief from the problem or from returning to health?

Check that you have not missed key symptoms and common disorders.
A few illnesses are particularly common among psychiatric inpatients and outpatients and therefore are often seen in psychiatric exams. If any of the characteristic symptoms listed here have not yet been considered, ask about them before leaving 'history of presenting complaints', just in case the patient has failed to mention their presence:
- **Low mood (depressive disorder).**
- **Elevated mood (bipolar affective disorder).**
- **Delusions and hallucinations (schizophrenia).**
- **Anxiety (generalized anxiety disorder).**
- **Panic attacks (panic disorder).**
- **Obsessional thoughts (obsessive– compulsive disorder).**

Other medical, psychiatric, and personal history

This section covers the remaining aspects of the history, including:

- Past psychiatric history.
- Past medical and surgical history.
- Medications and allergies.
- Alcohol and smoking.
- Illicit drugs.
- Family history.
- Premorbid personality.
- Personal history.

Often, one or more of these areas are of particular relevance to one or more of the presenting complaints and the details will have already been recounted in the history of presenting complaint. For instance, a patient who complains of having depression despite having tried three different antidepressants should have had their previous psychotropic drug usage recounted in the history of presenting complaint section. To avoid unnecessary repetition, only the present regimen should be presented here.

Past psychiatric history

Past psychiatric history consists of details of previous psychiatric illnesses prior to, or independent of, the episodes described in history of presenting complaint. This includes significant events such as suicide attempts, admission to inpatient units, outpatient contact with psychiatric services, and presentations in primary care with psychiatric symptoms. Dates and estimation of the severity and course of illnesses should be recorded.

Past medical and surgical history

Make a list of any significant medical illnesses or surgical procedures, with dates. It is worth enquiring specifically about head injuries, epilepsy, and endocrine abnormalities, given their relevance to psychiatric disorders.

Medications and allergies

It is good practice to list all medications the patient is using, both psychotropic drugs and those prescribed for non-psychiatric conditions, along with dose and regimen. Use of over-the-counter medications (e.g. codeine, laxatives) should also be recorded. Non-compliance with prescribed drugs should be noted here, as should adverse reactions and allergies.

Alcohol and smoking

Current intake of alcohol (in units) and smoking should be recorded here, along with previous smoking and drinking habits. If use of alcohol is high, consider the possibility of a dependence syndrome.

Illicit drugs

All patients should be asked whether they have used illicit drugs. Record the drug names, and the years and frequency of use.

Standard questions on suicidal ideas and previous attempts, illicit-drug use, forensic history, and sexual history should never be avoided for fear of adding to risk or offending the patient. However, with older patients in particular, sensitivity and discretion may be required in asking such questions.

Family history

It is important to record whether parents or other first-degree relatives (siblings, children) have suffered psychiatric illnesses (including suicide), especially as there is a genetic component in the risk of developing many psychiatric conditions. It may also be worth enquiring about physical illnesses (e.g. diabetes, myocardial infarction) that have affected first-degree relatives or the cause of death in any who have died.

Personal history

The personal history consists of a description of the patient's life, including:

- Birth (including complications).
- Childhood development and events, early childhood illness, contact with child psychiatrists.
- Brothers and sisters (it is customary to draw a small 'family tree' showing the patient's place in the family in relation to older and younger siblings).
- Relationship with parents.
- School (educational qualifications and other achievements, age on leaving, popularity, truancy and exclusions).
- Further education.
- Employment and work record.
- Relationships, marital and sexual history.
- Children (number, with sex, age, and any notable problems listed).
- Social situation (housing, members of household, contact with friends or family, involvement in hobbies).
- Financial situation.
- Forensic history (cautions, convictions, and time spent in prison).

Premorbid personality

The premorbid personality is an indication of the patient's personality before the development of psychiatric symptoms. The main purpose of this is to identify specific personality disorders and personality traits that may be predisposing factors for specific psychiatric illnesses (see Chapters 8 and 22).

MENTAL STATE EXAMINATION

After the history but prior to formulation, the mental state examination should be conducted. Just as a physical examination consists of inspection, palpation, and other specific tests involving percussion and auscultation, the mental state examination involves observations about the patient, direct questions, and, finally, specific tests (e.g. of registration and memory). When recording abnormalities noted in verbal sections of the mental state examination, it is often useful to illustrate the finding by quoting the patient's speech verbatim.

The mental state examination includes the following points.

Appearance

Regarding appearance, issues to consider include:

- Is the patient dressed conventionally or inappropriately (e.g. a manic episode may lead to selection of inordinately bright colours)?
- Do they appear dishevelled (may indicate alcohol problems, depression, or schizophrenia) or excessively thin (anorexia nervosa or depression)?
- Is there any evidence of self-harm (e.g. multiple cuts to wrists or forearms)?
- Are there obvious signs of a physical disorder?
- Is any other aspect of the appearance unusual (e.g. raw skin on hands in compulsive hand washing)?

Behaviour

It is usual to include a reference to the quality of the rapport and the patient's eye-contact with you. Most patients are co-operative and cordial, but sometimes patients may be:

- Reluctant to co-operate.
- Disinterested.
- Aggressive.
- Disinhibited (e.g. in manic episodes or schizophrenia).

There are no strict rules about the time period to which the mental state examination applies. It is not solely a snapshot of the present time. Although observations of behaviour and cognitive tests may reflect current function, areas such as mood and thought-content can take account of recent variations.

You may wish to take account of any relevant information relating to development of presenting symptoms (e.g. 'Recurrent worries about son over past 2 months which have subsided since his return 3 days ago').

When reassessing the patient, record details of the mental state in the period since the last assessment.

- Over-familiar with the interviewer.
- Agitated or distressed.
- Preoccupied (e.g. with obsessional thoughts or the content of delusions or hallucinations).
- Unresponsive (see Chapter 14).

When abnormal behaviour is detected, try to think through reasons why the patient is adopting that behaviour.

Abnormal movements

Abnormal movements may be associated with schizophrenia, neurological disease, or side effects of medications, and should be recorded.

Speech

The patient's speech should be assessed for:
- Speed and amount (pressure or poverty of speech).
- Spontaneity.
- Volume.
- Abnormalities in flow (e.g. stuttering).

'Poverty of content of speech' may be recorded when speech is understandable and adequate in amount but conveys little useful information as it is vague or contains many repetitions and obscure or stereotyped phrases.

Mood and affect

Both the patient's (subjective) estimation of mood and the interviewer's (objective) assessment should be recorded. The objective assessment relies on a fusion of the observations made about the patient's posture, facial expression, emotional reactivity, speech, and verbal clues to mood, in the interview so far. The subjective assessment is performed by asking directly how the patient is feeling, and if low mood is detected the presence of cognitive features (e.g. hopelessness, worthlessness, and guilt) may be elicited.

The distinction between mood and affect is discussed in Chapter 1. Affect may be:
- Blunted—the patient is unable to externalize happiness and sadness fully.
- Flat—little or no emotional reactivity.
- Labile—rapid changes are experienced and expressed.
- Incongruent or inappropriate—the patient's statements about their mood are quite different from that observed by the interviewer.

In addition to low or elevated mood the presence of features such as anxiety, fear, anger, or suspiciousness should also be assessed.

Suicidality

If not already established, the existence of suicidal ideas, plans, and intent should be determined and recorded here.

Thought-form

The term 'thought-disorder' describes a collection of abnormalities which may be noted in speech or writing but appear to reflect a fundamental disturbance in the process of formulating and expressing thoughts, i.e.:
- Tangentiality.
- Circumstantiality.

- Concrete thinking.
- Loosening of associations (including derailment and word salad).
- Blocking.
- Neologisms.
- Flight of ideas (including clang associations).

As these are abnormalities of thought-form rather than of thought-content, the phrase 'formal thought disorder' is often used. These features are closely associated with psychotic episodes (in schizophrenia or the manic phase of bipolar affective disorder) and are defined in Chapters 1 and 5.

When deciding whether formal thought disorder is present, you may need to make judgements based on the patient's speech and other forms of communication. For instance, flight of ideas and loosening of associations can be inferred from speech and are often accompanied by pressure of speech, while interruptions in speech may represent blocking. Recording a patient's words verbatim can be useful when thought disorder is suspected.

Thought-content

It is necessary to record here the details of any thoughts that frequently enter the patient's mind or represent specific disturbances in thought-content. Unless the area has been largely covered already, it is usual to start with an open question such as: 'Are there any worries or other things that you keep thinking about?'.

Closed questions can subsequently be used to elicit information on remaining aspects of thought-content. Features to enquire about include:
- Regular worries and preoccupations.
- Ruminations (repeated reflection back over an event or issue—these may meet the criteria for obsessional thoughts but are also encountered in generalized anxiety disorder and depressive episodes).
- Overvalued ideas (see Chapters 4 and 5).
- Obsessional thoughts (see Chapter 4).
- Phobias (see Chapter 3).
- Delusions (see Chapter 5).

If delusions are suspected, it is essential to establish their content and whether they are primary or secondary (e.g. to an abnormal mood state or to hallucinations). There are many further questions that can be asked: e.g. 'Do you feel that anyone might be planning to harm you?' (persecutory delusions); 'Do you consider yourself to have any special powers?' (grandiose delusions). A full discussion of how to elicit delusions can be found in Chapter 5.

Abnormal perceptions

It may be evident from the history that a patient has recently experienced hallucinations, and behaviour during the interview might also be suggestive of distraction by auditory or visual hallucinations. If hallucinations have not yet been discussed or noted, the interviewer should ask about them here.

When hallucinations are believed to be present, it is necessary to establish by further questioning:
- What is the content of the abnormal perception (e.g. threatening voices)?
- Are the abnormal perceptions true hallucinations, illusions, or pseudohallucinations?
- For hallucinations, which sensory modalities are involved (visual, auditory, olfactory, gustatory, bodily sensations)?
- In auditory hallucinations, does the perception come from inside or outside the head? Is there one voice or many? Is the first, second, or third person used? Do they involve the patient's own thoughts being echoed aloud (thought-echo) or a running commentary?
- If visual, is the image complex (e.g. a person) or simple (e.g. flashes of light)?

Derealization and depersonalization (see Chapter 9) should be recorded here.

Cognitive tests

Cognitive tests are discussed fully in Chapter 5. The main categories are:
- Orientation and consciousness.
- Attention and concentration.
- Memory.
- General knowledge and intelligence.

Insight

This final section of the mental state examination should involve an assessment of the patient's insight. This includes:
- Belief of being ill (and recognition of the illness as 'physical' or 'mental').
- Understanding of the illness.
- Recognition of the need for treatment.
- Willingness to accept treatment.

TERMINATING THE INTERVIEW

When bringing a psychiatric interview to a close, it is polite to thank the interviewee for their time and co-operation. As a medical student, it is worth remembering the following further points:

- Although discussions with staff members are to be encouraged, never discuss the patient by name with anyone who is not professionally involved—breaches of confidentiality can be disastrous in psychiatry.
- Transference and countertransference can occur (see Chapter 16).

THE FORMULATION

The history and mental state examination parts of a psychiatric assessment usually provide a wealth of information which must be utilized in order to make conclusions about diagnosis, aetiology, management, and prognosis. A formulation covers all these areas and is a crucial component of any assessment. Typically, the formulation is broken down into the following headings:

- Case summary.
- Differential diagnosis.
- Aetiology.
- Management—investigations, treatment.
- Prognosis.

To illustrate these points, an elaborated version of the 'psychotic patient' described in Chapter 5 will be used.

Case summary

The case summary comprises a few sentences recording the salient features of a case. Particular attention is paid to:

- Demographic details.
- Main components of history of presenting complaint.
- Significant background details, e.g. family history.
- Positive findings in the mental state examination.

Example

Mr DH is a 23-year-old, single, unemployed gentleman who was recently admitted under Section 2 of the Mental Health Act. He presented with a 6-month history of bizarre beliefs relating to being subject to government experiments and hearing voices through television and radio. In this time he has become more socially isolated and has terminated his job. He has no past psychiatric history but has an older brother with schizophrenia. On mental state examination he appeared unkempt and behaved suspiciously, demonstrating delusional beliefs of persecution, passivity, and thought-insertion following a delusional perception. He also demonstrated functional third-person hallucinations and appeared to have no insight into his illness.

Differential diagnosis

Deciding on the diagnosis can be a daunting task when given a lot of relatively unstructured information during an interview; a clear case-summary makes the task easier, although it can narrow down the differential too much.

It would be advisable to:

- Consider as wide a differential as possible, listing them in order of preference.
- Consider supporting and non-supporting evidence for each differential.
- Actively apply the classification hierarchy as a 'diagnostic sieve' so that important disorders are not missed (Fig. 14.2).
- Remember that two or more disorders can coexist, e.g. depression and alcohol dependence; in this event, try to decide if one is primary or secondary to the other, or whether they are independent.

Example

Mr DH's differential diagnosis.

Primary diagnosis:

- Schizophrenia—more than 1 month of symptoms: first-rank symptoms of delusional perception, passivity, thought-insertion, and third-person hallucinations. During this period there was also a

> The term 'neurotic' has largely fallen into disuse among modern classification systems. ICD-10 retains the term to broadly categorize phobic, anxiety, and obsessive–compulsive disorders. It is best avoided in exams.

decline in his personal functioning, and he had no insight into his illness.

Differential:
- Affective psychosis—either manic or depressive episode with psychotic features, but on mental state examination his mood was mainly suspicious as opposed to lowered or elevated, and appeared secondary to his delusional beliefs.
- Psychotic disorder induced by psychoactive substances—unlikely due to length of symptoms and his denial of alcohol and illicit substance use, but his symptoms may be exacerbated by covert substance use.
- Organic disorder—although rare in this age group, an early presenile dementia (e.g. Huntington's disease) or an organic psychosis should be excluded.

Although considered, there is insufficient evidence at this stage to support a comorbid diagnosis of a neurotic disorder, behavioural syndrome, or personality disorder.

Aetiology
The origins of most psychiatric disorders are thought to be multifactorial and, with the exception of organic disorders, can only, at best, be postulated for individual cases. However, this is an important part of the formulation as it helps develop a broader understanding of a case, to guide management and prognosis.

Example
Mr DH, primary diagnosis schizophrenia.
    Examples of possible aetiological factors for Mr DH's disorder are listed in Fig. 14.3.

Management
Investigations
Investigations should be justified on the following grounds:
- Helping to test and clarify the differential diagnosis.
- Excluding organic causes for the disorder.
- Excluding comorbid physical illness which might complicate the course and treatment of the psychiatric disorder.
- As a baseline measure prior to specific treatment, e.g. antipsychotics, lithium.

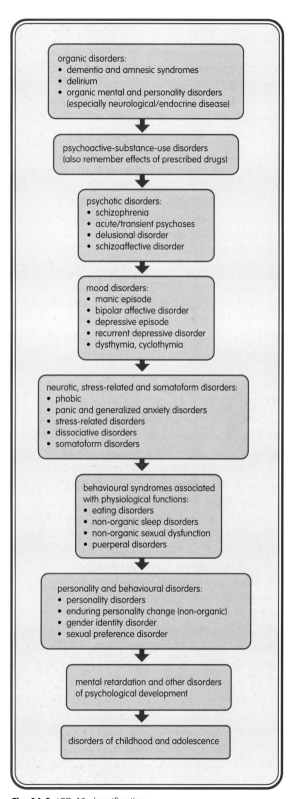

Fig. 14.2 ICD-10 classification.

103

Investigations may be further categorized into the following:
- Getting a corroborative history.
- Physical examination.
- Physical investigations.

Obtaining a corroborative history

A corroborative history is particularly important if the patient lacks insight through psychosis or cognitive dysfunction. All aspects of the history should be reviewed, especially premorbid personality as this is difficult to judge from a patient's subjective account. Sources of information include relatives, friends, the family doctor, and old notes. More specialist court, probation, and social-work reports may sometimes be available.

Physical examination

It is customary to carry out a full physical examination whenever a patient is admitted, although it is rarely performed in an outpatient setting. Areas to concentrate on are:

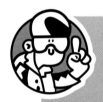

It is useful to think in terms of biological, psychological, and social aetiological factors and how these might predispose, precipitate, or perpetuate a disorder (the '3 Ps'). Combine individual factors specific to a case with the known aetiological causes for a specific disorder (see Fig. 14.3).

- Evidence of substance misuse, e.g. changes in pupil size, intravenous needle marks, signs of alcohol-related liver disease.
- Evidence of neurological or endocrine disease which may cause psychological symptoms, e.g. signs of raised intracranial pressure, thyroid eye disease.
- Evidence of psychotropic-drug-induced side effects (see Chapter 15), e.g. parkinsonism, tardive dyskinesia, hypotension.

Physical investigations

Physical investigations are usually performed when there is evidence from the history, mental state examination, and physical examination to suggest an underlying or comorbid organic disorder. Specific investigations for each disorder are listed, where relevant, in Part III, Diseases and Disorders.

In addition, physical investigations are usually indicated in the following circumstances:
- First presentation of a psychotic or severe mood disorder.
- Known comorbid physical illness (e.g. diabetes) or substance misuse.
- Atypical presentation, e.g. isolated auditory hallucinations in the absence of other psychopathology.
- Treatment resistance or intolerance.

Possible aetiological factors for Mr DH's disorder			
Factor	**Biological**	**Psychological**	**Social**
predisposing	family history of schizophrenia	—	—
precipitating	? amphetamine use 6 months ago reported by sister	—	separation from partner and change of address 8 months ago
perpetuating	—	plans to return to 'high expressed emotion' family environment	lack of other social supports, unemployment

Fig. 14.3 Possible aetiological factors for Mr DH's disorder.

Example

After a full physical examination, and a corroborative history from his parents and family doctor, Mr DH was further investigated with:

- Full blood count (FBC)—to exclude excessive alcohol use, baseline prior to antipsychotics.
- Urea and electrolytes (U/Es)—to exclude renal and endocrine disease.
- Thyroid function tests.
- Calcium—to exclude renal and endocrine disease.
- Glucose—to exclude diabetes and hypoglycaemia.
- Liver function tests—to exclude alcohol misuse, baseline prior to antipsychotics.
- Erythrocyte sedimentation rate (ESR)—to exclude inflammatory cause of psychosis.
- Urine drug screen—to exclude illicit-substance use causing or potentiating psychosis.
- Electroencephalogram (EEG) or computerised tomography (CT) scan—may be considered to exclude an organic disorder.

Treatment

As with aetiology, it is useful to think in terms of biological (e.g. drugs, electroconvulsive therapy, psychosurgery), psychological (e.g. counselling, psychotherapy) and social (e.g. occupational, housing assistance) approaches. Each can be further divided into short-term, medium-term, and long-term treatments.

Example

Mr DH, primary diagnosis schizophrenia (Fig. 14.4).

Prognosis

The prognosis is dependent on two considerations:

- The natural course of a disorder based on studies of patient populations; these are discussed for each disorder in Part III, Diseases and Disorders.
- Individual factors pertaining to the patient in question, e.g. social stability, and compliance with treatment.

In an exam, ensure you can justify any physical investigations on clinical grounds.

Example

Assuming Mr DH has a diagnosis of schizophrenia, it is likely his disorder will run a chronic course, either relapsing/remitting or persistent symptoms +/− decline in personal functioning. Approximately 20% have no further relapses after recovery, although the long onset and course of his symptoms, social isolation, and single status point to a poorer prognosis.

Possible treatment options for Mr DH			
Term	**Biological**	**Psychological**	**Social**
short (hours–days)	establish antipsychotic drugs	try to build rapport with patient, assess suicide/dangerousness risk carefully	deal with immediate problems, e.g. source of income, debts
medium (days–months)	consider depot if problems with compliance	as insight develops, provide further advice for patient and carers	assess for care programme approach, consider involving community psychiatric nurse and/or social worker
long (months–years)	review treatment according to clinical response	consider specific family interventions	assist rehabilitation to independent accommodation and work

Fig. 14.4 Possible treatment options for Mr DH.

THE LONG CASE EXAM

The long case exam usually involves an hour-long interview with an unknown patient followed by a presentation to examiners. It assesses history taking, mental state examination, and the ability to make a formulation. Although an artificial situation, it is modelled on everyday clinical work, so the best preparation is to see plenty of patients!

Preparation
On the day, it is advisable to:
- Arrive early, bring spare pens and plenty of paper.
- Dress conservatively—it is likely examiners will be.
- Write down all headings for each area of history, mental state, and formulation, so important parts are not forgotten.

Patient interview
You will be nervous at the patient interview. Explain to the patient why you are interviewing them and warn that you may need to interrupt or redirect the conversation because of the time limits. Also explain that you will be asking many 'standard' questions, exploring background as well as current details. The order you take the history is unimportant providing you cover all the headings—ask the patient directly what their diagnosis and treatment are. Try to complete the interview in under 50 minutes, giving yourself at least 10 minutes to work through the formulation. As you work through the formulation it is best to keep the patient with you so you can ask anything you may have forgotten.

Presentation
Anxiety causes people to speak faster, therefore consciously speak more slowly when presenting the case; headings should be spoken clearly, followed by a pause, to keep the attention of examiners.

The presentation should take about 10 minutes; the history of presenting complaint and mental state should take about a third of this time each. If the patient is a poor or vague historian, explain to the examiners beforehand (thinking why this might be so) and concentrate more efforts on the mental state.

Finish with a summary of the case and ensure you are prepared for questions on the other aspects of the formulation.

THE SHORT CASE EXAM

In some clinical exams students are presented with either a short video of a patient, or an actor presenting as a patient – both of which last approximately ten minutes. In the former, the student is asked to comment on the patient's mental state, and perhaps suggest a differential diagnosis. In the latter, the student is asked to elicit some aspect of the 'patient's' history or mental state, and perhaps give feedback on diagnosis, treatment, or prognosis. This is one of the most daunting of all clinical exams in that an examiner is usually present, and time is at a premium.

Useful advice includes:
- Try to suspend disbelief at the unreality of the situation, treat the 'patient' as if they were real.
- *How* you elicit the information is just as important as *what* information you obtain. The examiners are looking for sensitive, empathic students who listen as well as question. Introduce yourself and your role, check the patient's name (avoid using their Christian name), seek permission to ask questions on the area instructed (e.g. 'I wonder if I could ask some questions relating to your mood?').
- Try to ignore the examiner(s). Avoid looking for feedback; tell the patient to ignore the examiner.
- Listen carefully to what the patient says. Try not to rush through your own agenda; clarify their terminology (e.g. 'I feel anxious'), attend to any clues which suggest psychopathology (e.g. 'I knew I was special when the police started following me') and reflect on what the patient says, (e.g. 'I've felt low ever since father died...'–reply: 'It sounds like that was a painful event for you...').
- Use open questions. You can interrupt if the patient digresses, e.g. 'That sounds like an important matter for you, perhaps we can come back to it at the end. Now I'd like to know about..'
- Practise interview skills with your colleagues. You should be able to elicit information regarding: abnormal mood, suicidal ideation, anxiety symptoms, obsessions, delusions, hallucinations, alcohol/drug history, and cognitive state examination.
- If asked to give feedback a degree of caution is acceptable, e.g. 'Although I would normally have had more time to ask questions, from what you have told me you may be suffering from depression at the moment'.

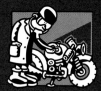

15. Pharmacotherapy and Physical Treatments

Antidepressants

Antidepressants (Fig. 15.1) are subdivided into three main classes:

- Tricyclic drugs (TCAs)—so called because of their three-ring chemical structure.
- Selective serotonin reuptake inhibitors (SSRIs)—named for their action on the neurotransmitter serotonin.
- Monoamine oxidase inhibitors (MAOIs)—named for their action on the presynaptic enzyme monoamine oxidase type A.

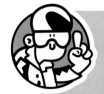

When revising the antidepressants, start by familiarizing yourself with the three main classes (tricyclics, SSRIs, and MAOIs), then learn the names of one or two drugs from each of the subgroups in Fig. 15.1.

Historical perspective

Antidepressants were first used in the late 1950s, with the appearance of the tricyclic agent imipramine and the monoamine oxidase inhibitor (MAOI) phenelzine.

The former class was enlarged throughout the 1960s and 1970s to more than ten tricyclics and related compounds. A major development in the 1980s was the arrival of the first selective serotonin reuptake

Fig. 15.1 Classification of antidepressants.

Classification of antidepressants			
	Tricyclics	**SSRIs**	**MAOIs**
'early' (late 1950s/early 1960s)	amitriptyline imipramine	—	phenelzine tranylcypromine isocarboxazid
'modern'	dothiepin lofepramine clomipramine trimipramine doxepin nortriptyline	fluoxetine paroxetine sertraline citalopram fluvoxamine	moclobemide (RIMA)
related compounds	trazodone mianserin reboxetine (NaRI) mirtazepine (NaSSA)	venlafaxine (SNRI) nefazodone (*)	—

Within each of the seven sub-groups the drugs are listed in order of total number of prescriptions in the UK for 1996.
RIMA: Reverse inhibitor of monamine oxidase
SNRI: Serotonin and noradrenaline reuptake inhibitor
* Serotonin reuptake inhibitor and 5HT1A inhibitor
NaRI: Noradrenaline re-uptake inhibitor
NaSSA: Noradrenergic and specific serotonergic antidepressant

inhibitors (SSRIs): fluvoxamine and fluoxetine (Prozac®). There has since been considerable expansion of the SSRI class, as well as a revival of the MAOIs through the development of the reversible MAOI moclobemide. Additional compounds related to the main classes have also appeared.

Indications

Tricyclic agents are used in the treatment of:
- Depression.
- Panic disorder.
- Obsessive–compulsive disorder (clomipramine).
- Post-traumatic stress disorder (imipramine and amitriptyline).
- Other conditions such as chronic pain and nocturnal enuresis.

SSRIs are used in:
- Depression.
- Panic disorder.
- Obsessive–compulsive disorder (fluvoxamine, sertraline, fluoxetine).
- Bulimia nervosa (fluoxetine).
- Social phobia (occasionally).

MAOIs are indicated for all types of depression, although historically they were preferred when atypical features such as excessive sleeping, overeating, and anxiety were present. They may also be effective in social phobia and other anxiety disorders.

Mechanism of action

In simple terms, all three classes of antidepressants act by increasing the amount of neurotransmitter present in the synaptic cleft (Fig. 15.2). Tricyclics achieve this by preventing presynaptic reuptake of the transmitter noradrenaline; SSRIs by preventing reuptake of serotonin. There is some overlap— tricyclics, especially clomipramine, do have some affinity for blocking serotonin reuptake.

MAOIs inhibit an enzyme in the presynaptic terminal which breaks down monoamines such as noradrenaline and serotonin, therefore making more neurotransmitter available for release. The newer drug moclobemide is a RIMA, the 'RI' indicating that it is a reversible competitive inhibitor of monoamine oxidase.

For these mechanisms of action to be valid, we must assume that an increase in the amount of monoamine (noradrenaline or serotonin) in the synaptic cleft has an

impact on depressive symptoms through postsynaptic effects. Such effects may be mediated by binding to membrane G proteins, causing activation of intracellular second-messenger systems, which may, over a period of weeks, induce subtle adaptations to key proteins.

Clinical considerations

Efficacy

Despite nearly 40 years of development, no antidepressant has been shown to have greater efficacy than any other (with the possible exception of venlafaxine—on the basis of small studies, greater efficacy at high doses has been claimed). Every agent, when prescribed correctly, should produce remittance of depressive symptoms in approximately 60% of patients within 4–6 weeks.

Doses and administration

One reason why antidepressants fail to produce their intended effect is because they are prescribed at doses too low for the therapeutic effect to occur. This is a particular problem with many tricyclics (including imipramine, amitriptyline, and lofepramine), for which a dose of greater than 125 mg per day is required in depressed subjects. Patients sometimes do get better on lower doses, but, until a drug has been prescribed at a 'therapeutic' dose for 6 weeks, it cannot be considered to have been given an adequate trial. SSRIs are more straightforward in this respect, most offering a simple 'one tablet a day' schedule (e.g. fluoxetine or paroxetine at 20 mg/day).

For panic disorder, lower starting doses are recommended, especially for SSRIs. Patients should be warned about the possibility of a 'jitteriness syndrome' over the first 2–3 weeks, in which free-floating anxiety may increase before panic attacks are eventually reduced.

When a patient using a tricyclic or SSRI is changed to one of the older MAOIs, and vice versa, the potential for drug interactions is such that there must be a washout period of 2 weeks (or as long as 5 weeks for the SSRI fluoxetine) between treatments. However, because of its short half-life, a washout period is not required when changing from the 'modern' MAOI moclobemide to another antidepressant.

When depressive symptoms have remitted antidepressants should be continued for 6 months, but for recurrent depressive disorder long term maintenance therapy may be required.

Side effects

As antidepressants all have a similar efficacy, the choice of which drug to prescribe often rests on their markedly different side effect profiles.

As well as having affinity for noradrenergic receptors, tricyclic drugs are known to act on muscarinic receptors, producing 'anticholinergic effects'. These unwanted side effects include:

- Dry mouth.
- Difficulty in micturition/urinary retention.
- Blurred vision.
- Constipation.

Tricyclic agents may also cause sedation. For a depressed person who continues to work in a job involving the performance of skilled tasks such as operating machinery, or who needs to drive, this may be highly undesirable. On the other hand, a severely depressed person who has given up work and driving may benefit immensely from a drug that improves a disturbed sleep pattern. Sedative tricyclics may be a good choice in depressed patients who are additionally anxious and agitated.

Weight gain is associated with tricyclics, but not with SSRIs.

There is some evidence that newer tricyclics such as lofepramine may cause significantly less frequent side effects than the original tricyclics imipramine and amitriptyline.

SSRIs were initially thought to be associated with fewer side effects than tricyclics, but recent analyses have thrown this claim into doubt. The first 'S' in their name implies that they are more selective for the serotonin receptor and have little affinity for the muscarinic receptor, hence avoiding the above anticholinergic effects. However, they are

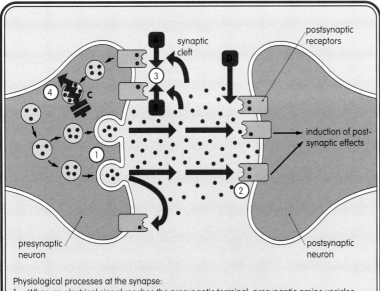

Fig. 15.2 Mechanism of action of antidepressants at the synapse.

Physiological processes at the synapse:
1. When an electrical signal reaches the presynaptic terminal, presynaptic amine vesicles fuse with the neuronal membrane and release their contents into the synaptic cleft.
2. Amines in the synaptic cleft bind to postsynaptic receptors to produce a post synaptic response.
3. Amines may be removed from the synaptic cleft by reuptake into the presynaptic neuron.
4. The monoamine oxidase enzyme breaks down presynaptic amines.

Effects of antidepressants:
A. Tricyclics mainly prevent presynaptic reuptake of nonadrenaline.
B. SSRIs predominantly block reuptake of serotonin.
C. MAOIs reduce the activity of monoamine oxidase in breaking down presynaptic amines (leaving more available for release into the synaptic cleft).
D. Some antidepressants (e.g. nefazodone) inhibit postsynaptic receptors directly.

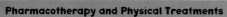

associated with a different group of side effects, including:

- Headache.
- Nausea.
- Gastrointestinal disturbance/diarrhoea.
- Abdominal pain.

The original MAOIs such as phenelzine and isocarboxazid fell out of favour, largely through the possibility of interactions with certain foods and other drugs. A patient using one of these MAOIs must be warned to avoid:

- Tyramine-rich foods.
- Cold remedies containing ephedrine.
- Other antidepressants.

Examples of foods rich in tyramine include:

- Cheese (especially mature cheeses like Stilton) and foods containing cheese (e.g. pizza).
- Chianti wine.
- Pickled herring.
- Broad-bean pods.
- Yeast extracts (e.g. marmite).
- Soya-containing foods.

If such warnings are not heeded, there may be a 'cheese reaction'. This dangerous event is heralded by a throbbing headache and, possibly, a stiff neck and sweating. If a hypertensive crisis develops, it may be treated by the calcium antagonist nifedipine. The newer drug moclobemide is much less likely to precipitate a cheese reaction and therefore dietary restrictions are limited, but patients should still avoid ephedrine-based drugs and large quantities of the tyramine-rich foods.

Like tricyclics, phenelzine and isocarboxazid may cause drowsiness, dry mouth, and blurred vision. Postural hypotension and dizziness may be a problem in the elderly. Moclobemide may promote agitation and initially can make sleep difficult.

Toxicity

Some tricyclics, notably dothiepin and amitriptyline and to some extent imipramine, are highly toxic in overdose, whereas lofepramine and trazodone are relatively safe. The former drugs cause cardiotoxicity through their ability to prolong the Q–T interval and it is generally better to avoid them in a patient expressing active suicidal ideation.

SSRIs are safe in overdose, although earlier concerns were expressed that prescription of fluoxetine to depressed patients might be associated with an increase in completed suicide through violent means. Large analyses have concluded that no such association exists and SSRIs can be prescribed with confidence to depressed patients expressing suicidal ideation.

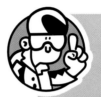

Amitriptyline, clomipramine, dothiepin, and trazodone are the most sedating of the commonly prescribed tricyclic and modified tricyclic drugs. Imipramine and lofepramine are much less sedating.

Antipsychotics (or 'neuroleptics')

Historical perspective

Antipsychotics (originally known as 'major tranquillizers' and then as 'neuroleptics') appeared at the end of the 1950s with the introduction of chlorpromazine. Their ability to treat schizophrenia and other psychotic disorders meant that they had a profound impact on psychiatry—in particular accelerating the movement of patients out of the old asylums and into the community. By the mid-1980s, a large range of antipsychotics was available, but it was the successful reintroduction of an old drug, clozapine, which has ushered in the appearance of a group of atypical antipsychotic agents in the 1990s.

Classification of antipsychotics

Antipsychotic agents (Fig. 15.3) were originally classified according to their structure alone (phenothiazines, butyrophenones, etc.), those in the phenothiazine group being subcategorized into type I, II, or III, with drugs in each subcategory having similar propensity to cause sedative, antimuscarinic, and

Classification and side effects of antipsychotics			
Conventional antipsychotics	**Sedation**	**Anti-muscarinic effects**	**Likelihood of EPSEs**
phenothiazines: type 1 (chlorpromazine, promazine)	+++	++	++
phenothiazines: type 2 (pericyazine, thioridazine)	++ or +++	+++	+
phenothiazines: type 3 (prochlorperazine, trifluoperazine)	+	+	+++
butyrophenones (haloperidol,droperidol) subst. benzamides (sulpiride) thioxanthines (flupenthixol, zuclopenthixol)	+	+	+++
atypical antipsychotics: • clozapine • risperidone • olanzapine • sertindole • quetiapine • amisulpride	++ + + 0 or + + +	+++ + + + + +	0 + 0 or + 0 0 0 or +

Fig. 15.3 Classification and side effects of antipsychotics.

extrapyramidal side effects. However, when clozapine returned to prominence, it was considered clinically distinct from other antipsychotics because of its lack of extrapyramidal side effects, and it was given the label 'atypical' in recognition of this difference. The existing antipsychotics were therefore labelled 'conventional'. Further drugs have been added to the atypical group, namely risperidone, which can cause extrapyramidal side effects but is different from the conventional psychotics in structure and receptor specificity, and olanzapine, sertindole, and quetiapine, which were designed to be similar in activity to clozapine and appear to be free of extrapyramidal side effects.

Indications
Antipsychotics are indicated for:
- Schizophrenia and schizoaffective disorder.
- Psychotic symptoms in depression and bipolar affective disorder.
- Severe anxiety and agitation (short-term use only).
- Gilles de la Tourette's syndrome (haloperidol, chlorpromazine).
- Amphetamine psychosis (haloperidol).
- Nausea and vomiting (perphenazine).

- Calming patients with an acute behavioural disturbance whatever the underlying cause.

Mechanism of action
There are many hypotheses about the cause of schizophrenia. Supporters of the 'dopamine hypothesis', which proposes that schizophrenia is associated with an excess of dopamine, believe that antipsychotics work by blocking CNS dopamine receptors—in particular the D_2 receptor. The dopamine hypothesis has been thrown into question by the fact that clozapine, an effective antipsychotic, has little or no affinity for the D_2 receptor, but is a strong antagonist of D_4 and 5-HT$_2$ receptors and has affinity for muscarinic, noradrenergic, and histaminergic receptors.

Thus it is likely that the antipsychotic effect of these drugs results from interaction with a number of receptor systems, particularly those of a dopaminergic (e.g. D_2, D_3 and D_4) and serotonergic nature.

Clinical considerations
Efficacy
Provided the antipsychotic is titrated up to an appropriate dose, over two-thirds of patients with schizophrenia or other psychoses should have some remission of their

symptoms, although in half of these, symptoms may recur despite ongoing treatment. Positive symptoms of schizophrenia are more likely to respond than negative, but atypical antipsychotics are more likely to treat negative symptoms than are conventional drugs.

Dose and administration

Owing to the variability of response and the potential for side effects, antipsychotics are initially prescribed at low doses, which can be titrated up to, or beyond, the maximum licensed dose (e.g. haloperidol may be started at doses of 2–5 mg twice daily, and increased incrementally to the maximum dose of 120 mg/day or beyond). Although high doses may calm acute behavioural disturbance, they are no more effective in treating underlying psychotic disorders than an 'optimal' range of lower doses. Whilst it is usual to start with a conventional antipsychotic in a newly diagnosed schizophrenic patient, atypical drugs may be introduced if extrapyramidal side effects develop or if there is no improvement with two conventional drugs (Fig. 15.4).

Some antipsychotics may be given intramuscularly, especially in acute behavioural disturbance. When acute psychosis produces an extreme behavioural disturbance, which may include violent resistance with potential danger to ward staff, the heavily sedating zuclopenthixol (Acuphase®) may be given by this route—patients must be observed carefully in the hours after it is given.

Conventional antipsychotics are also available as slow-release 'depot' preparations. Depots can be given intramuscularly every 2, 3, or 4 weeks as maintenance therapy for patients with psychotic disorders in remission, eliminating the need to take daily tablets and the potential for poor compliance.

Side effects

Side effects of antipsychotics include:

- Sedation—this is the most common side effect of antipsychotics and occurs in the majority of patients, being most pronounced with type I phenothiazines (e.g. chlorpromazine).
- Extrapyramidal side effects—these movement disorders are a neurological consequence of antipsychotic usage and are summarized in Fig. 15.5. Parkinsonian symptoms, akathisia, and dystonia tend to appear within days of starting treatment (although akathisia can be difficult to differentiate from the symptoms of the underlying illness). Each of these

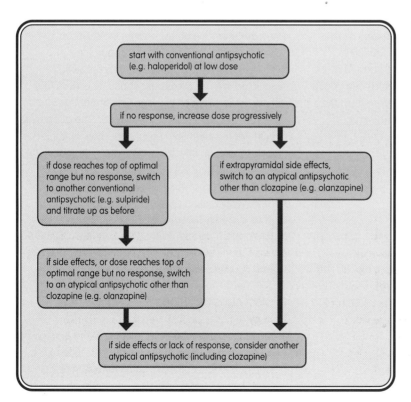

Fig. 15.4 A typical protocol for the administration of antipsychotics to a patient newly diagnosed with schizophrenia.

symptoms can be combated by the introduction of antimuscarinic agents such as procyclidine or orphenadrine, and should subside if the antipsychotic is stopped, although akathisia may respond only if Parkinsonian symptoms are also present. Tardive dyskinesia, however, takes much longer to develop, is not amenable to treatment with antimuscarinic drugs (which may make it worse), and may be irreversible, persisting when the antipsychotic is stopped.

- Antimuscarinic side effects—occurring in one-third of patients on conventional antipsychotics, these side effects are similar to those evoked by tricyclic antidepressants (see page 109) and include dry mouth, constipation, and urinary retention. The effects may be exacerbated by antimuscarinic drugs introduced to combat extrapyramidal side effects.

- Postural hypotension—some antipsychotics, including chlorpromazine, thioridazine, and all the atypical drugs, block α-adrenoceptors and may cause postural hypotension; the patient feeling dizzy on standing up, and sometimes fainting. Such falls may cause physical damage, notably in the elderly. Fortunately, tolerance soon develops.

- Weight gain—this may occur to excess with many conventional antipsychotics, especially fluphenazine and flupenthixol; atypical drugs, including clozapine, are also associated with weight gain.

- Prolactin levels—all conventional antipsychotics and some atypicals raise prolactin levels as a consequence of dopaminergic blockade and may cause galactorrhoea and menstrual disturbances in women.

- Seizures—antipsychotics may lower the convulsion threshold; chlorpromazine, thioridazine, and clozapine carry the greatest risk.

- Cardiac arrhythmias—most antipsychotics prolong the Q–T interval and may theoretically predispose to ventricular arrhythmias. An ECG is required before using sertindole or prescribing any antipsychotic beyond the maximum licensed dose.

Description of extrapyramidal side effects	
Extra-pyramidal side effect	**Description**
Parkinsonian symptoms	muscular rigidity, cogwheeling and tremor similar to that seen in Parkinson's disease
akathisia	motor restlessness, especially of legs, causing a subjective inability to relax
dystonia	abnormal movements of facial muscles or the tongue. The eyes may be affected producing oculo-gyric crisis
tardive dyskinesia	variety of abnormal movements ranging from minor tapping to facial grimacing and on to twisting and gyrating of the body

Fig. 15.5 Description of extrapyramidal side effects.

Patients on the atypical antipsychotic clozapine are at risk of haematological effects such as neutropenia and the life-threatening agranulocytosis. The drug must be started in hospital and a monitoring service provided. Blood samples must be taken weekly for 4 months, then fortnightly; only when counts have been stable for at least a year is the frequency cut to every 4 weeks.

Despite the need for such active monitoring, clozapine is widely used in patients with treatment-resistant schizophrenia, owing to its improved efficacy over conventional drugs for negative symptoms and its reduced potential for extrapyramidal side effects.

Toxicity

The neuroleptic malignant syndrome is a rare but life-threatening complication of neuroleptic usage. Symptoms and signs include:

- Fluctuating consciousness.
- Sweating and high temperature.
- Muscular rigidity/dystonia.
- Tachycardia.
- Elevation of blood pressure.

If the syndrome is recognized, neuroleptic medication should be stopped and dantrolene (a drug used in the treatment of malignant hyperthermia) or bromocriptine (a dopamine agonist) may be administered.

Antipsychotics with strong anticholinergic effects, especially when prescribed in combination with antimuscarinic agents, may provoke central antimuscarinic toxicity, leading to memory loss, confusion, and hallucinations. Fortunately, this syndrome is usually reversible on stopping treatment.

Lithium and other mood-stabilizing agents

Mood-stabilizing agents include:

- Lithium salts (e.g. lithium carbonate).
- Carbamazepine.
- Sodium valproate.

Lithium

Historical perspective

Although lithium salts had been known as a constituent of medicinal spa waters in Victorian times, it was a chance discovery by the Australian Cade in 1949 which pointed to its potential value as a mood-stabilizing agent. Trials in the 1950s and 1960s led to the drug entering mainstream practice in 1970.

Indications

Lithium has two main indications:

- Prophylaxis and treatment of bipolar affective disorder, including treatment of acute manic episodes.
- Treatment of depressive disorders resistant to treatment with conventional antidepressants. In this case lithium is prescribed in combination with an existing tricyclic or SSRI ('lithium augmentation').

Mechanism of action

The mechanism of action of lithium remains a mystery. It may work through blocking the inositol phosphatase second-messenger system as it is known to inhibit a number of steps in this pathway.

Clinical considerations

Efficacy

Lithium is effective in the prophylaxis and treatment of 50–75% patients with bipolar affective disorder. When introduced to treat an acute manic episode, it is often prescribed in combination with an antipsychotic agent for the first 3 weeks because its onset of action may be delayed.

When lithium is used to augment antidepressive treatment in patients with recurrent depression, it may be effective in 50% of patients who have not responded to an antidepressant alone.

Dose and administration

Lithium has a narrow 'therapeutic window' between the blood level at which therapeutic benefits may be gained and the level at which toxic effects may be expected. Its kinetics are relatively simple—it is eliminated unchanged by the kidney and its half-life is affected by renal function and therefore increases with age. Before starting lithium therapy, the following blood investigations should be performed:

- Urea and electrolytes (in addition to renal function, the lithium plasma level is influenced by sodium depletion).
- Thyroid function tests.
- Full blood count.

Monitoring of lithium blood levels is essential but easily undertaken. Samples are usually drawn in the morning, 12 hours after the last evening dose.

Lithium is normally taken twice daily. The drug should be started at a low dose which depends on the actual preparation used, so trade names (e.g. Camcolit®, Priadel®) are always stated when prescribing lithium. A blood sample should be taken when this steady state is established (at least 1 week later); the dose may then be titrated upwards until the blood level comes within the safe therapeutic range of around 0.5–1.0 mmol/l (the exact range is subject to local variations). Once lithium has been established at an appropriate plasma level, the patient should be advised to return at intervals of approximately 4 months for further blood monitoring, with adjustment of the dose as required.

Side effects

As lithium, even when levels are in the therapeutic range, may provoke a host of side effects, patients should always be educated regarding adverse effects. A treatment card documenting possible side effects should be handed out before commencing treatment so that an informed choice can be made by the patient regarding pros and cons of lithium therapy.

Potential side effects include:
- Fine tremor, especially of the fingers.
- Gastrointestinal disturbance.
- Polyuria and polydipsia.
- Weight gain.
- Goitre and hypothyroidism.
- Arrhythmias and ECG changes.

Toxicity

Toxic effects may result from a lithium plasma level greater than 1.5 mmol/l. Initial signs of lithium toxicity are tremor, marked gastrointestinal disturbance (including diarrhoea and vomiting), dysarthria, and ataxia, followed by muscle fasciculations, loss of consciousness, and seizures. In such circumstances, lithium should be stopped and sodium-containing fluid should be given to reverse the toxicity.

Carbamazepine and sodium valproate

Carbamazepine may be familiar as a first-line agent in the treatment of epilepsy, but it may also be used for prophylaxis in bipolar affective disorder where lithium has failed or has caused intolerable side effects. It is effective in approximately 60% of patients and appears to be especially useful when bipolar illness is 'rapid cycling' (four or more manic or depressive episodes per year).

Potential side effects of carbamazepine include:
- Gastrointestinal disturbance.
- Dizziness.
- Double vision.
- Leucopenia.
- Pruritic rash.
- Raised liver enzymes.

The last three of these side effects occasionally lead to more dangerous complications—respectively, aplastic anaemia, exfoliative dermatitis, and hepatitis.

Sodium valproate, another drug commonly used in epilepsy, may also be of benefit in prophylaxis of bipolar affective disorder.

Benzodiazepines
Classification

Benzodiazepines may be classified according to their structure, by their indication, or as short-acting or long-acting compounds (Fig. 15.6).

Historical perspective

In the 1960s the benzodiazepines replaced the barbiturates as drugs of choice for the treatment of anxiety and insomnia. The great initial enthusiasm for these drugs, however, was tempered by the finding that they were associated with addiction and withdrawal syndromes. Today benzodiazepines are widely used but with much more caution to avoid a time-limited prescription for transient symptoms being inadvertently continued, potentially leading to a long-term addiction.

Indications

The indications for individual benzodiazepines are summarized in Fig. 15.6.

Benzodiazepines are used in:
- Insomnia—short-acting benzodiazepines (e.g. temazepam) have the advantage of causing no hangover effect on the following day, but are more likely to be associated with withdrawal effects. The drugs should be prescribed on a time-limited basis, and may be more effective if taken on alternate nights rather than nightly, to reduce the chance of tolerance developing.
- Anxiety—diazepam and lorazepam are regularly prescribed in generalized anxiety disorder. Benzodiazepines are also used to control anxiety symptoms occurring in adjustment disorders and may also be given to a person who is experiencing pronounced but transient symptoms in the face of a sudden stressor (e.g. a road accident) when no psychiatric diagnosis applies. Alprazolam has been used successfully to control panic attacks in patients with panic disorder, and to relieve symptoms in individuals with social phobia. Again, in view of the potential for addiction or difficult withdrawal, the

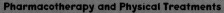

Classification of benzodiazepines				
Benzodiazepine	Structure	Insomnia	Anxiety	Alcohol withdrawal
short-acting drugs				
temazepam	3-hydroxy benzodiazepine	√		
lorazepam	3-hydroxy benzodiazepine	√	√	
oxazepam	3-hydroxy benzodiazepine		√	
alprazolam	triazolo benzodiazepine		√	
long-acting drugs				
diazepam	2-keto benzodiazepine	√	√	
flurazepam	2-keto benzodiazepine	√		
chlordiazepoxide	2-keto benzodiazepine		√	√
nitrazepam	2-keto benzodiazepine	√		√

Fig. 15.6 Classification of benzodiazepines.

drugs are usually given at low doses for limited periods, although a patient with chronic generalized anxiety may require maintenance therapy. Note that, unlike antidepressants, benzodiazepines produce their desired effect quickly and tablets may used as required (PRN) as 'rescue medication' when severe anxiety is experienced.

- Alcohol withdrawal—chlordiazepoxide (or occasionally diazepam) may be used as an adjunct in alcohol withdrawal. At the start of detoxification, alcohol intake is replaced by prescribed benzodiazepines, which are gradually reduced over a period of 7–10 days. Chlormethiazole (see page 118) is an alternative to benzodiazepines for this purpose.
- Mixed anxiety and depressive conditions— benzodiazepines are prescribed along with antidepressants when depressive disorders are associated with significant anxiety symptoms.
- Non-psychiatric indications—certain benzodiazepines are used in epilepsy; clonazepam has antiepileptic action, and diazepam and other compounds are indicated in the emergency management of status epilepticus.

Mechanism of action

Benzodiazepines exert their action by binding to a site associated with the $GABA_A$ receptor which is linked to a chloride ion channel. The action of the inhibitory neurotransmitter GABA is enhanced.

Clinical considerations

Dose and administration

The potency of the benzodiazepines varies across the class, so that 5 mg of diazepam is equivalent to just 1 mg of lorazepam. The drugs are usually taken orally, but diazepam and lorazepam may be given intramuscularly for control of severe anxiety. Furthermore, intravenous infusion of benzodiazepines may be undertaken in the management of status epilepticus and severe acute behavioural disturbance.

Side effects

Although the sedative effect of benzodiazepines is useful in the treatment of insomnia, drowsiness is commonly a problem when they are used for other indications, and patients need to be warned about the potential dangers of driving or operating machinery. Benzodiazepines depress brain respiratory centres and must be used with caution in patients with chronic respiratory disease. They may also cause dizziness or akathisia, especially in elderly patients.

Withdrawal syndrome

Factors that make benzodiazepine withdrawal syndromes more likely to occur are:
- Prolonged use.
- Short-acting rather than long-acting drug.
- High dose and/or abrupt discontinuation (the dose should be tapered).

Withdrawal symptoms may occur up to 3 weeks after stopping benzodiazepines. Up to 40% of benzodiazepine users may experience one or more of the following symptoms:
- Anxiety, depression, and paranoia.
- Tremor.
- Loss of appetite.
- Perspiration.
- Tiredness.
- Irritability.
- Depersonalization or perceptual disturbance.

Toxicity

When an overdose of benzodiazepines alone is taken, the outcome is generally good, although respiratory depression and loss of consciousness can occur. Combinations of benzodiazepines with other substances that potentiate their action (e.g. alcohol or antidepressants) may be much more dangerous.

Other hypnotic and anxiolytic agents

See Fig. 15.7 for a classification of other hypnotic and anxiolytic agents.

Chloral hydrate has been available for over 100 years. Its use is now limited, but it may be used to control insomnia for very short periods (2–3 days), most often in children and young adults. It causes gastric irritation and may provoke arrhythmia in overdose and so should be avoided in suicidal patients.

The hypnotics zopiclone and zolpidem are innovations of the 1990s. Although structurally different to benzodiazepines, they are thought to act at the same receptor. Like temazepam, they have a short half-life and therefore do not cause a hangover on the following day. They should be used for limited periods only. Suggestions that they are not associated with dependence or early tolerance, and that zolpidem in particular produces sleep architecture more similar to natural sleep than do benzodiazepines, should be treated with caution given that these drugs are still relatively new.

Buspirone, a $5-HT_{1a}$ receptor antagonist, is another new drug which may be used in place of benzodiazepines for the management of anxiety disorders. It does not sedate and is not thought to be associated with dependence, addiction, or withdrawal phenomena, but it takes longer to produce its therapeutic effect. It is safe in overdose, but common side effects include headache, nausea, and dizziness.

Fig. 15.7 Classification of other hypnotic and anxiolytic agents.

Classification of other hypnotic and anxiolytic agents				
Drug name	Structure	Insomnia	Anxiety	Alcohol withdrawal
chloral hydrate	$CCl_3CH(OH)_2$	√		
zolpidem	imidazoppyridine	√		
zopiclone	cyclopyrrolonene	√		
buspirone	azaspirone		√	
chlormethiazole	thiazole derivative	√		√

Chlormethiazole is structurally related to vitamin B_1 and may be used in alcohol detoxification, but is not the first-choice agent. Due to a potential for respiratory depression, it may be dangerous if a patient leaves the programme and takes large quantities of alcohol whilst continuing the drug. There is also a potential for dependence. For these reasons it is given on a reducing course lasting 7–9 days, after which no more is made available.

Antimuscarinic, anticholinergic, or antiparkinsonian agents

Antiparkinsonian drugs, including procyclidine, orphenadrine, and benzhexol, act on muscarinic acetylcholine receptors. As well as being indicated for patients with Parkinson's disease, they are widely used in psychiatry to counteract extrapyramidal movement disorders related to antipsychotic drugs.

When a newly diagnosed schizophrenic patient is prescribed a conventional antipsychotic such as haloperidol, parkinsonian symptoms (rigidity, cogwheeling, tremor, etc.), dystonias, or akathisia may soon develop. An antimuscarinic agent such as procyclidine can be added to the regimen, usually on a PRN basis, to be taken until the symptoms are suppressed. However, routine administration of antimuscarinic agents when antipsychotics are first prescribed is unwise, as they may alter the absorption of the antipsychotic and may even make tardive dyskinesia more likely to develop.

Blockade of muscarinic receptors may produce a similar set of side effects to those encountered with tricyclic antidepressants, including blurred vision, urinary retention, and even the provocation of narrow angle glaucoma in vulnerable patients.

Other drugs used in psychiatry

Several other pharmacological treatments are used in psychiatry—most in subspecialties. For example:

- Donepezil, a reversible anticholinesterase inhibitor, is given for mild or moderate dementia in Alzheimer's disease, where it is believed to slow the progression of deterioration (see Chapter 17).
- Alprostadil, a prostaglandin, is used for the treatment of erectile dysfunction (see Chapter 22).
- Beta-blockers such as propanolol may provide relief of autonomic symptoms in anxiety disorders. The β-blocker pindolol may be effective as an adjunct to

SSRIs in the treatment of depression.
- Disulfiram may be initiated to help chronic alcoholics give up their habit (see Chapter 18).
- Methadone is used as a replacement treatment in patients with opioid dependence and naltrexone is an opioid antagonist useful in relapse prevention. Lofexidine is an alpha receptor agonist useful in opioid withdrawal (see Chapter 18).
- Methylphenidate, an amphetamine analogue, is used in child psychiatry to treat hyperkinetic disorder (see Chapter 24).

Why do psychotropic drugs fail?

A drug failure occurs when a prescribed medication does not produce an adequate therapeutic effect. This may simply reflect a resistance of the individual's symptoms to the actions of the drug, but several other explanations should be considered:

- The patient may have been misdiagnosed (e.g. a patient with schizophrenia misdiagnosed as having bipolar affective disorder is much less likely to respond to lithium).
- An apparent psychiatric disorder may be entirely secondary to an undiagnosed organic disorder which requires treatment (e.g. anxiety secondary to hyperthyroidism).
- The dose of the psychotropic agent may have been too low.
- The drug may have been given for too short a period.
- Efficacy may have been impaired by an interaction with another drug—prescribed or unprescribed.
- The patient may have poor compliance because of unpleasant side effects, poor motivation, lack of initial response, or a regimen that is unreasonably complicated. Some may even have resolved not to take the drug at all. Non-compliance can be reduced by good patient education, but some non-compliers will insist they have taken a drug as instructed for fear of offending the clinician—only drug plasma levels can demonstrate non-compliance with certainty.

Drug indications

Indications of the major groups of psychotropic drugs are summarized in Fig. 15.8. Remember that psychiatric illnesses are often associated with comorbid conditions which may themselves require treatment—for example, schizophrenia may be associated with depression, so both antipsychotics and antidepressants may be required.

Summary of psychotropic drug indications					
	Antidepressants	Lithium	Antipsychotics	Benzodiazepines	Other hypnotic and anxiolytic drugs
depressive disorders	√	√1			
bipolar affective disorder		√	√2		
depressive disorders with psychotic symptoms	√	√1	√		
generalised anxiety disorder			√3	√	√4
panic disorder	√			√	
phobias	√5				
obsessive–compulsive disorder	√6	√7			
post-traumatic stress disorder	√8				
schizophrenia			√		
acute behavioural disturbance			√	√	
alcohol withdrawal				√	√9
insomnia	√10			√	√
eating disorders	√11				

Key: √recognised indication
1. Lithium is given in combination with tricyclic or SSRI antidepressants, usually when symptoms have proved resistant to treatment with adequate doses of two or more antidepressants.
2. Antipsychotics are often used to treat acute manic episodes.
3. Antipsychotics may be used for the short term management of severe anxiety.
4. Buspirone may be used in generalized anxiety disorder as an alternative to benzodiazepines.
5. Phenelzine (MAOI) is effective in social phobia, as may be SSRIs.
6. The tricyclic clomipramine and the SSRIs fluvoxamine, sertraline and fluoxetine are effective in treatment of obsessive–compulsive disorder.
7. Lithium augmentation is occasionally tried when obsessive–compulsive disorder is resistant to antidepressant treatment.
8. There is evidence that tricyclics (especially imipramine and amitriptyline) and SSRIs may be effective in post traumatic stress disorder.
9. Chlormethiazole is an alternative to benzodiazepines in alcohol withdrawal.
10. When a patient complaining of insomnia also has depression, a sedative tricyclic antidepressant such as trazodone or amitriptyline should be considered. SSRIs do not provide rapid sedation in such patients but may improve the quality of sleep over a longer period.
11. Fluoxetine is licensed for the treatment of bulimia nervosa.

Fig. 15.8 Summary of psychotropic drug indications.

PHYSICAL TREATMENTS

Electroconvulsive therapy
Historical perspective
Electroconvulsive therapy (ECT) was first used systematically in the 1930s, after observations that seizures induced by camphor could temper the symptoms of depression and schizophrenia. Seizures were originally administered without anaesthesia, but this changed in the 1950s with the development of suitable short-acting anaesthetics and muscle relaxants. Although numerous drug treatments have arrived over the last 40 years, ECT has remained as an alternative strategy, especially for patients resistant to drug therapy.

Indications

Although ECT is normally reserved until trials of appropriate drugs have failed, it is as effective as pharmacotherapy for:

- Major depression.
- Bipolar affective disorder.

It is also occasionally used in:

- Acute episodes of schizophrenia (especially those with positive symptoms or catatonia).
- Obsessive–compulsive disorder.

Administration

Before commencing a course of ECT, a patient should have a documented physical examination, an ECG, and blood tests including full blood count, and urea and electrolytes. Informed consent is needed (except when ECT is performed under the provision of the Mental Health Act). The patient must avoid food and drink on the morning before therapy.

Electroconvulsive therapy is performed in theatre, with an anaesthetist on hand to administer a general anaesthetic, oxygen, and muscle relaxants. A charge, preset by the operator on the basis of the patient's sex, height, weight, and any previous ECT settings, is delivered to the scalp via electrodes placed unilaterally or bilaterally. The desired goal is a bilateral fit involving the whole body and lasting from 15 to 35 seconds.

Patients are often drowsy when woken from anaesthesia after treatment. They are taken to a recovery room and observed. Those being given ECT on an outpatient basis must be warned not to drive for the rest of the day and, if possible, should be accompanied home by a family member or friend.

Side effects

As in any procedure that requires anaesthesia, the effects of the anaesthetic and its administration (e.g. dental damage on intubation) are risks associated with ECT therapy.

Transient memory loss is the most commonly reported side effect of the ECT itself. Cardiac arrhythmias have also been reported.

Psychosurgery

Psychosurgical procedures (such as prefrontal leucotomy) were prevalent in the 1930s and 1940s, despite the surgeons of the day lacking modern stereotactic techniques that allow lesions to be localized precisely. Psychosurgery is rarely used in present-day practice, but operations may occasionally be undertaken in patients with chronic depressive disorders or certain persistent anxiety disorders, including obsessive–compulsive disorder.

Modern-day operations using stereotactic techniques include:

- Limbic leucotomy.
- Tractotomy.
- Amygdalotomy.

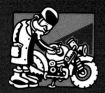

16. Psychotherapy and Service Provision

Psychological treatments are frequently used in the management of psychiatric disorders, either as the treatment of choice or to augment physical treatments.

Psychotherapy may be defined as a treatment that manages psychological symptoms by using the professional relationship between a patient and a therapist to change feelings, cognition, and behaviour.

At the heart of all psychological treatments is the empathic communication between the therapist and the patient which involves—to varying degrees—listening, talking, emotional expression, interpretation, and advice.

Patients undergoing psychotherapy may be seen individually, with partners, with their family, or as part of a larger group. The 'therapist' can include any health worker with expertise in psychotherapy, and psychiatrists with a special interest in this field may train to become consultant psychotherapists.

Supportive psychotherapy and counselling

Counselling services are widespread within the voluntary sector, primary care, and large employers. Practices vary, but the general approach is to provide relatively brief interventions to people with a variety of psychological symptoms and life stresses. The counselling approach developed by Carl Rogers— client-centred psychotherapy—assumes a passive, non-directive role for the therapist, who accepts and reflects on whatever the patient says, in order to build a therapeutic relationship.

Supportive psychotherapy builds upon the basic tenets of all psychotherapy, but is more directive in nature, involving reassurance and advice. The aim is to develop a supportive relationship so that patients feel comfortable to discuss their current problems and feelings with a non-judgemental professional. An essential component in everyday consultations for all doctors, supportive psychotherapy therefore has universal application to psychological problems, whether they are short-term stress or intractable personality disorders.

The main specialist psychotherapies and their theoretical bases will now be considered in turn.

Psychodynamic psychotherapy

Psychodynamic psychotherapy is distinguished by the emphasis given to the resolution of unconscious conflicts as a means of changing undesirable thoughts and feelings, using the relationship between the therapist and the patient as a key mechanism to effect this change.

It is a broad term which encompasses several different theoretical approaches and practices. Each of these can be traced back to the influential ideas of Sigmund Freud, whose theories of the mind led to the practice of psychoanalysis.

To understand the practice of psychodynamic psychotherapy, it is worthwhile considering some of the basic psychoanalytic concepts.

Topographical model

In the topographical model, the mind has both unconscious and conscious psychological processes; the former is not readily accessible to consciousness, consisting of instinctual drives (e.g. sexual, aggressive), ideas, and memories.

Structural model

The structural model is a refinement of the above. It divides the mind into the:
- Id (child-like)—a wholly unconscious collection of inborn drives.
- Superego (parent-like)—a partly conscious and partly unconscious set of ideals which form an individual's conscience through childhood development.
- Ego (adult-like)—a partly conscious and partly unconscious agency which mediates between the demands of the id, the demands of external reality, and those of the superego.

Developmental model

Individuals pass through several stages of development in early life, during which unconscious drives come into conflict with external reality. During these stages, individuals are vulnerable to external stresses and this can lead to problems in later life through incomplete resolution of these conflicts. (Freud named the stages Oral, Anal, Phallic, Latent, and Genital.) For example, consciousness represses unpleasant memories of sexual abuse into the unconscious, but the associated emotional energy persists and is prone to break through into consciousness at other times—through psychiatric symptoms.

Defence Mechanisms

Unpleasant unconscious impulses, memories, or emotions are prevented from reaching consciousness by employing defence mechanisms. Many defence mechanisms have been described, including:

- Denial—closely related to the process of repression discussed above, the individual lacks awareness for something they should know, e.g. death of a loved one.
- Projection—the individual attributes their own thoughts and feelings to another to make them more palatable, e.g. the cheating husband develops intense jealousy of his wife.
- Dissociation (conversion)—unpleasant thoughts or feelings manifest as cognitive symptoms (e.g. memory loss) or physical symptoms (e.g. paralysis). This concept remains highly influential and is the basis for the dissociative (conversion) disorders (see Chapter 9).
- Sublimation—unacceptable thoughts or impulses (e.g. aggression) are diverted into socially acceptable activities such as sport or hobbies.

Defence mechanisms are not necessarily abnormal and are employed by everyone at some stage of their lives; for example, denial is considered a normal stage in grief reactions.

Transference and Countertransference

Transference is the name given to the patient's transfer to the therapist of feelings associated with their early relationships. These feelings may be positive or negative, depending on the situation, e.g. a male patient becomes angry with the therapist who he sees as cold and uncaring, unconsciously reminding him of his mother. Likewise, therapists develop a countertransference towards patients

during therapy, based on their own life experiences, and this can be dangerous to patients if communicated openly, e.g. expressing outright anger and hostility towards suicidal patients. It is important to note that psychoanalysts would expect transference and countertransference relationships to develop in all therapeutic settings.

Psychodynamic Therapy in Practice

Freud's ideas have been developed by others in the last 100 years, most notably by Carl Jung (Analytical Psychology) and Melanie Klein (Object Relations School). Most psychodynamic therapists now incorporate a variety of psychoanalytic theories.

The general principles of psychodynamic therapy are:

- The therapist remains passive, i.e. does not give explicit advice on how to alleviate symptoms, but helps the patient to work through unconscious conflicts rather than offering specific solutions.
- Unconscious conflicts are identified by interpretation of defence mechanisms, dreams, parapraxes (slips of the tongue—'Freudian slips'), and psychological symptoms. 'Free association' is the method developed by Freud to help isolate unconscious processes—the patient is asked to say spontaneously whatever comes into his head.
- Particular attention is given to identifying and interpreting the significance of transference and countertransference feelings. In long-term therapy these can reach intense proportions and the therapeutic relationship is usually governed by strict boundaries; e.g. sessions occur only at specified times and for a specific length, therapists do not divulge any personal information, and therapists are closely supervised by peers.

Cognitive and behavioural psychotherapy

In recent decades, cognitive and behavioural psychotherapy have gained increasing importance in the treatment of mental disorder. Abnormal thoughts and behaviours are considered to derive from dysfunctional patterns of learning, therefore greater emphasis is given to environmental aetiological factors. Behavioural therapy largely arises from theories of associative learning, whereas cognitive therapy largely arises from cognitive models of learning.

Associative learning

Two principle forms of associative learning are recognized, based on animal models:

- Classical conditioning (Pavlov, dog experiments)—an unconditioned stimulus (meat) causes an unconditioned response (salivation); a conditioned stimulus (bell) is repeatedly given with the unconditioned stimulus, to produce the unconditioned response; eventually, the conditioned stimulus alone gives rise to the conditioned response (salivation).
- Operant conditioning (Skinner, rat experiments)—independent of a stimulus, a behaviour recurs because it is positively reinforced, e.g. the rat learns to step on a lever to obtain food. This is otherwise known as trial-and-error learning, and behaviours may be discouraged by negative reinforcers.

Cognitive learning

Cognitive learning is the term given to the process whereby information is received, processed, and organized into cognitive structures, so enabling an individual to make sense of his or her world. Mechanisms involved include:

- Observation and imitation of others (observational learning).
- Sudden insights into problems (insight learning).

Social learning theory

By combining elements of associative and cognitive learning theory, social learning theory asserts that an individual's attitudes and behaviour are shaped by the society within which they develop, through the process of socialization.

Behavioural therapy

Behavioural therapy begins with a functional analysis—a careful history concentrates on the 'problem behaviour', dividing it into a chain of antecedents→behaviours→consequences (ABC). For example, in a patient with a spider phobia:

- A—encounters with spiders, thoughts of spiders, images of spiders on television or in books.
- B—symptoms of anxiety, need to escape the situation.
- C—avoidance of situations where spiders may be found, e.g. gardens.

Asking a patient to keep a diary of these events is often helpful; this can later be incorporated to measure treatment success.

Some of the behavioural treatments are described below.

Exposure

Exposure therapy is useful for tackling phobias and compulsive rituals. There are two approaches:

- Systematic desensitization—the patient is gradually exposed to the feared stimulus by progressing through a hierarchy of severity, e.g. patient made to think of spider→spider in same room as patient→spider near to patient→spider on patient's hand.
- Flooding—the patient is suddenly exposed to the feared stimulus with support from the therapist. Flooding in the imagination is known as implosion.

Relaxation training

Relaxation techniques promote gradual relaxation of muscle groups with neutral or pleasant mental imagery to alleviate anxiety. It may be used alone for anxiety management, or as an adjunct to other behavioural and cognitive techniques.

Response prevention

This technique is often combined with exposure techniques in the treatment of compulsive rituals: it requires constant staff persuasion and reassurance to prevent the undesired behaviour.

Social skills/assertiveness training

Training in social skills or assertiveness uses techniques such as role playing and modelling (where behaviour is shaped towards that of another) in group situations.

Behaviour Modification

The principles of operant conditioning can be utilized to shape desired behaviour in a variety of clinical settings, e.g. challenging behaviour among the learning disabled, difficult behaviour in children, and negative symptoms in schizophrenics. Desired behaviour is reinforced and rewarded, e.g. using gifts or tokens ('token economy') which are removed if undesired behaviour occurs.

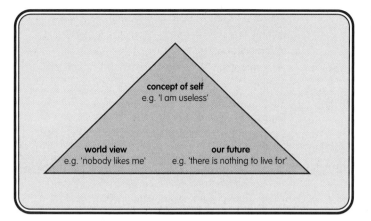

Fig. 16.1 Cognitive triad (with depressive cognitions).

concept of self
e.g. 'I am useless'

world view
e.g. 'nobody likes me'

our future
e.g. 'there is nothing to live for'

Cognitive therapy

Cognitive therapy developed from the work of Aaron Beck in the 1960s and 1970s. Initially concentrating on depression, he contended that recurrent faulty cognitions lay at the heart of this disorder. During childhood, a number of basic assumptions develop which enable us to build a (subjective) reality of our inner and outer worlds. They form a cognitive triad (Fig. 16.1).

From dysfunctional basic assumptions, cognitive distortions arise (i.e. a tendency to distort or misconstrue situations)—e.g.:

- 'He ignored me; it just shows nobody loves me' (overgeneralization).
- 'Passing my finals doesn't prove anything' (minimization).

Assessment of patients for cognitive therapy attempts to carefully extricate and identify these recurrent thought patterns. Use of a diary to record thoughts and feelings in given situations is again useful. Once identified, the thoughts are challenged by the therapist, and the patient is given help to counteract them.

Techniques used in cognitive therapy include:

- Distraction—focusing attention on other thoughts or the external environment.
- Thought stopping—a specific treatment for obsessional thoughts, the patient must try to switch their thoughts to another topic by using a sudden stimulus (e.g. snapping rubber band on their wrist) or making a noise (e.g. shouting 'stop!').
- Patient taught to develop rational responses to abnormal thoughts.

In practice, cognitive and behavioural approaches are usually combined as cognitive–behavioural therapy (CBT).

Applications of psychotherapy
Indications

Cognitive–behavioural therapy is now used in most types of psychiatric disorder, as listed in Fig. 16.2.

Psychodynamic therapies have a less well demarcated 'menu' of disorders which would benefit from this approach. Brief interventions may be useful for adjustment reactions or time limited disorders such as a single episode of depression. Longer interventions may be required for recurrent mood disorders, chronic anxiety disorders, and personality disorders. This approach is generally unsuitable for psychotic disorders or patients with seriously impulsive behaviour (e.g. substance abuse, borderline personality disorder).

Efficacy

Compared with the evaluation of drug treatments, it is more difficult to perform analogous large-scale randomized clinical trials of psychological therapies. The evidence to date indicates at least equal efficacy of psychological treatments compared with drug treatments for certain disorders; for example, cognitive–behavioural therapy of mild or moderate depressive disorders is as efficacious as antidepressants. Unsurprisingly, better results occur with more-experienced therapists.

Patient characteristics

The specialized psychotherapies are both time consuming and potentially demanding. It may be extremely unpleasant to confront phobias or deal with unpleasant childhood memories. For both cognitive–behavioural and psychodynamic therapies, patients should be carefully assessed beforehand to judge their motivation and capacity to work psychologically.

A comparison of psychodynamic and cognitive–behavioural therapies is shown in Fig. 16.3.

Applications of cognitive–behavioural therapies	
Disorder (main applications)	**Methods used**
depressive (mild–moderate)	relaxation social skills/assertiveness challenge cognitive distortions
panic, phobic and generalized anxiety disorders	exposure (to anxiety provoking situations) relaxation challenge cognitive distortions
obsessive–compulsive disorder	exposure (to anxiety provoking situations) response prevention modelling thought stopping
learning disability (behaviour problems)	behaviour modification

Other disorders where CBT may be used

dementia	post traumatic stress disorder
chronic psychosis	eating disorders
bereavement reactions	sexual dysfunction
somatization disorder	substance misuse
personality disorder	child behaviour problems

Fig. 16.2 Applications of cognitive–behavioural therapies.

MENTAL HEALTH LEGISLATION AND SERVICE PROVISION

This section of the chapter will outline:
- The legal framework for the treatment of the mentally disordered.
- Historical trends in service provision and recent developments in community care.

The details apply specifically to the United Kingdom.

Consent to treatment

In order to get a patient's consent, a doctor is obliged to explain in general terms, the reasons for, the nature of, and the likely risks and benefits of, the treatment—this consent can subsequently be withdrawn by the patient at any time. There are, however, occasions when a patient is unable to give valid consent: if the patient is unconscious, has cognitive dysfunction, or has impaired judgement secondary to a psychosis.

Under Common Law, doctors are allowed to deliver both medical and psychiatric treatments

Comparison of psychodynamic and cognitive–behavioural therapies		
Feature	**Psychodynamic**	**Cognitive–behavioural**
therapist	passive, interprets unconscious processes, non-directive, interested in early life relationships and their influence on symptoms	active, directive, does not interpret unconscious processes, interested in current behaviour and thoughts
length of treatment	usually long term (>6 months) but brief forms occur	usually short term (<6 months) with specified number of sessions
settings	individual, marital, family, group	usually individual, sometimes groups
goal of treatment	develop insight into problems, work through dysfunctional patterns of relating to others	relieve symptoms and change existing patterns of undesirable behaviours

Fig. 16.3 Comparison of psychodynamic and cognitive–behavioural therapies.

without informed consent when failure to do so would lead to death or severe harm to the patient or others, e.g. in cases of hypoglycaemic coma or delirium. In addition to short-term treatment of medical or psychiatric emergencies, Common Law enables longer-term treatment of 'incompetent' patients, such as those with severe learning disability or dementia.

Many anomalies emerge: for example, Common Law would not authorize the amputation of a 'competent' person's gangrenous leg even though the procedure is life saving. In general, doctors err towards treatment when the patient is deemed incompetent of valid consent—if ever unsure, it is wise to contact seniors or defence organizations.

The issue of consent to treatment is particularly important for psychiatrists, given that a substantial proportion of mentally disordered patients frequently lack insight into their illness and would pose a risk to themselves or others if left untreated. At the same time, patients require specific rights under the law so that they are not detained and treated indiscriminately.

The Mental Health Act

The Mental Health Act of 1983 (England and Wales) provides a detailed legal framework for the detention, treatment, and discharge of mentally disordered patients in hospital. It is divided into 10 Parts, each of which is further divided into Sections.

Definition of mental disorder

Part I of the Mental Health Act categorizes four types of mental disorder:

- Mental illness—this is not defined by the Act and is left to clinical judgement. In practice, this term covers the majority of disorders encountered in psychiatry, except for personality disorders and learning disability, which are developmental rather than acquired.
- Psychopathic disorder—this is defined as 'a persistent disorder or disability of mind (whether or not including significant impairment of intelligence) which results in abnormally aggressive or seriously irresponsible conduct on the part of the person concerned'. Among psychiatrists it is a controversial and rarely used category (except in forensic settings); clinically it best approximates to severe dissocial and borderline personality disorders.

- Mental impairment and severe mental impairment—these definitions combine learning disability and psychopathic disorder.

The Act does not cover other behaviour which may be deemed 'undesirable', e.g. promiscuity or substance misuse—unless there is a comorbid mental disorder.

The Mental Health Act is an example of Statutory Law, which is formed through an Act of Parliament. Common Law refers to law developed by the judiciary through historical precedent.

Detention under the Mental Health Act

To detain a patient in hospital under a Section, the following criteria must be satisfied:

- The patient suffers from a mental disorder as defined by the Act.
- The patient presents an immediate risk to themselves, either directly as a result of self-harm or indirectly as a result of a deterioration of their disorder.
- The patient presents an immediate risk to others.
- The risks would be safeguarded by admission to hospital.

For most Sections, at least one of the recommending doctors should be approved under Section 12 of the Act. Approval is usually granted to psychiatrists who have completed their MRCPsych or other doctors with more than 3 years' experience.

Similarly, Approved Social Workers (ASWs) are social workers with special training enabling them to administer the Act.

The important Sections of Part II of the Act ('civil sections') are summarized in Fig. 16.4. For patients involved in criminal proceedings, Part III of the Act is applied—this is discussed briefly in Chapter 26.

Treatment provision under the Mental Health Act

The Act only authorizes compulsory treatment for the mental disorder itself (e.g. psychotropic drugs, psychotherapy, occupational therapy) or conditions directly resulting from the mental disorder (e.g. nasogastric feeding for anorexia nervosa). It does not authorize other medical treatments for the medically ill—irrespective of whether they have a mental disorder. Therefore, the depressed patient refusing acetylcysteine for a paracetamol overdose can only be treated medically under Common Law.

If a patient on a Section 3 withholds consent to treatment after 3 months, a second opinion appointed doctor (SOAD) must assess the patient to authorize further compulsory treatment. He or she is an experienced psychiatrist appointed by the Mental Health Act Commission (MHAC).

The situation regarding special treatments is as follows:

- ECT—if a patient withholds consent, an SOAD is required at any time to authorize compulsory treatment. It may be given urgently, without either consent or a second opinion, if the patient's life

Sections of Part II of the Mental Health Act 1983 enabling compulsory admission					
Section	**Application and recommendations**	**Duration**	**Treatment**	**Discharge/Renewal**	**Notes**
2 admission for assessment	applicant: ASW or nearest relative recommendation: 2 doctors, at least one approved	28 days	may be given compulsorily	patient must appeal during first 14 days. May be discharged by RMO, MHRT, hospital managers or nearest relative	useful when diagnosis and likely response to treatment are unknown. If a longer period of detention is required, it is converted to a 3 before expiry
3 admission for treatment	applicant: ASW or nearest relative recommendation: 2 doctors, at least one approved	6 months	may be given compulsorily during first 3 months, after this time a second opinion is required to give treatment without consent	patients can appeal at any time. May be discharged during the section by their RMO, MHRT, hospital managers or nearest relative	this order is applied when the diagnosis is established and a clear treatment plan is known. For psychopathic disorder and mental impairment the proposed treatment must alleviate the condition or prevent deterioration
4 emergency admission for assessment	applicant: ASW or nearest relative recommendation: any doctor	72 hours	with consent or under Common Law only	no rights of appeal, only RMO can discharge	used infrequently and only recommended when the need for admission overrides any delay incurred waiting for the second medical opinion
5(2) doctor emergency holding order	one medical recommendation: the RMO or his nominated deputy	72 hours (patient is already admitted to hospital)	with consent or under Common Law only	no rights of appeal, only RMO can discharge	the order is designed to keep patients in hospital until a Section 2 or 3 can be completed
5(4) nurse emergency holding order	one recommendation from a registered mental nurse	6 hours (patient already being treated informally for a mental disorder)	with consent or under Common Law only	no rights of appeal, it lapses when the doctor arrives, he then has to decide whether a 5(2) is appropriate	used only when it is not possible to have the patient assessed by a doctor

Fig. 16.4 Sections of Part II of the Mental Health Act 1983 enabling compulsory admission.

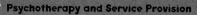

would be at risk otherwise, e.g. in cases of depressive stupor.
- Psychosurgery/hormone implants—these can be given only with the patient's informed consent and the support of an SOAD. Ability to consent is verified by a panel from the MHAC.

Appeals
All patients detained under Sections 2 and 3 may appeal through:
- The hospital managers directly.
- A Mental Health Review Tribunal (MHRT)—this usually consists of a lawyer, a lay-person, and an independent psychiatrist, who hear reports from the RMO and ASW. Patients may be represented by solicitors.

The law in Scotland
The law in Scotland was formalized by the Mental Health (Scotland) Act 1984. Psychopathic disorder does not appear, although a similar description is defined under the category of mental illness. The compulsory admission and treatment procedures are similar to those for England and Wales, although detention for longer than 28 days requires a successful application to the local Sheriff. Appeals are heard by the Sheriff or Mental Welfare Commission for Scotland.

The law in Northern Ireland
The Mental Health (Northern Ireland) Order 1986 also resembles the 1983 Act in its treatment and detention provisions. However, it excludes psychopathic (and personality) disorder.

Service provision
Historical perspective
Until the 18th Century, care for the mentally ill was almost entirely in the community, and many frequently fared no better than criminals or vagrants. With the industrial revolution and growth of cities, new legislation paved the way for specialist hospital provision. By the late 19th Century, all parts of Britain were served by large asylums, each housing many patients in self-contained communities.

Inpatient numbers peaked in the mid-1950s and have fallen dramatically since. The cause of this decline is multifactorial and includes the following:
- Economics—hospital care is very expensive.

- Development of effective drug treatments—especially antipsychotics.
- Concern over civil liberties of patients incarcerated for long periods.
- Recognition of damaging institutionalization among long-stay patients—apathy, loss of life-skills, inability to adapt.

Community care
Although the care of the mentally ill has shifted to the community over the last 40 years, the term 'community care' has gained popularity only since the early 1980s, when it became the focus of successive health and social service policy. It is, nevertheless, a vague term which covers a host of multidisciplinary services. The main components of most services for adult mental health are described below.

Primary care
General practitioners see the majority of mental disorder—largely mild affective and anxiety disorders.

Acute inpatient units
Acute inpatient units are organized at a district level and are designed to admit patients with an episode of a more severe disorder (psychotic, major affective, substance misuse) where community care is not feasible, e.g. to prevent self-harm, to contain disturbed behaviour, to supervise treatment.

Rehabilitation services
Rehabilitation services provide longer-term admissions and aftercare for patients whose social and living skills are severely handicapped by the effects of their illness (most commonly schizophrenia).

Day hospitals
Day hospitals serve a variety of functions; for example, they may provide alternative acute care for patients who would normally have been admitted to inpatient wards, or intensive treatment programmes for more severe non-psychotic disorders (e.g. obsessive–compulsive disorder, generalized anxiety).

Community mental health centres
Community mental health centres provide more-accessible services to local communities, enabling

assessment of new patients and crisis intervention. They act as a base for a number of professionals; of particular importance are Community Psychiatric Nurses (CPNs), who fill a number of important roles:

- Assessing urgent referrals.
- Monitoring patients in the community.
- Administering medication and providing psychological treatments.
- Coordinating other services, e.g. housing, social services, voluntary services.

Voluntary organizations
Both national (e.g. MIND, SANE) and local groups exist providing extensive advice and support for patients and carers. Some organizations provide supported accommodation and day centres.

Disadvantages of community care
Patients generally prefer to be treated out of hospital, and psychiatric bed numbers continue to decline; however, there are potential drawbacks to the current trend:

- It is often difficult for acutely ill patients to gain admission to hospital when they need to, and they may be inadequately prepared on discharge.
- A significant minority of chronically ill patients require ongoing hospital care or intensive community support but often languish on acute wards ('new long-stay').
- Patients frequently have a poor quality of life in the community because of stigmatization, unemployment, inadequate housing, and limited coping skills.
- Patients frequently become socially isolated and easily drift away from services.
- The need for multiple agencies to provide services (e.g. health, social, and voluntary services) can lead to fragmented care.

Several measures have been introduced to help solve some of these problems and thus improve community care.

Section 117 of the Mental Health Act has always provided a legal right to aftercare (by health and local authorities) for detained patients. Additional measures have been introduced recently, and these are reviewed below.

Care-programme approach (CPA) 1990
The key elements of the CPA are:

- A written care plan.
- A named keyworker (usually a CPN, social worker or consultant) to coordinate services and act if the care plan is not working.
- Regular reviews which include all relevant professionals, the patient, and carers.

All patients seen by psychiatric services should be screened for the CPA. Most districts divide the patients into tiers according to their needs. The elements described above are usually implemented in patients who:

- Require frequent admissions to hospital for chronic, often disabling, disorders.
- Tend to become disengaged from services and fail to seek help when their illness relapses.
- Require several services, e.g. social work, housing, CPN.
- Are a high risk to themselves or others as a result of their illness.

Supervision register 1994
Each health district is obliged to keep a central register of patients considered to pose a high risk of harm to themselves (through suicide or self-neglect) or considered dangerous to others. In addition to the provisions of the CPA, these patients are obliged to have more intensive contact with their keyworker and regular risk assessment.

Supervised discharge 1996
In addition to the above, supervised discharge facilitates immediate review of the patient by the keyworker, with powers to convey the patient to a health centre for further assessment; admission and treatment without the consent of the patient still requires use of the existing Mental Health Act.

129

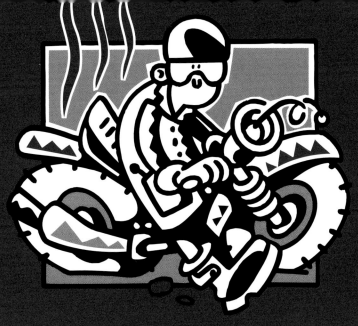

DISEASES AND DISORDERS

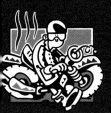

17. Dementia and Delirium

As dementia and delirium represent two distinct clinical syndromes, each will be considered separately. Diagnosis and clinical assessment are covered in Chapter 6.

DEMENTIA

The diagnostic criteria for dementia are listed in Fig. 17.1.

Aetiology

The neuropathology and clinical presentations of the main types of dementia are described in Chapter 6. Again, it is necessary to separate each type owing to their distinct aetiological factors.

Alzheimer's disease

Genetic factors

Family studies show a threefold increased risk of developing Alzheimer's disease in first-degree relatives of sufferers. Some families show an autosomal dominant pattern of inheritance for the disease. Adults with trisomy 21 (Down syndrome) always develop Alzheimer's disease pathology by middle age.

In recent years, several genes have been linked to the disease:

- Chromosome 21—amyloid precursor protein gene (re: trisomy 21, increased amyloid precursor protein production); this is particularly linked with rare familial cases.
- Chromosome 19—apolipoprotein E gene; the allelic variant $\varepsilon 2$ is protective, whereas the allelic variant $\varepsilon 4$ increases risk (homozygotes 8×, heterozygotes 3×).
- Chromosome 14—presenalin 1 gene.
- Chromosome 1—presenalin 2 gene.
- Chromosome 12—recent linkage with late-onset cases.

Environmental factors

There is no consistent evidence to confirm the role of toxins, viruses, and autoimmune factors in the aetiology of Alzheimer's disease. Aluminium is related to Alzheimer's disease pathology in dialysis patients, but it has not been shown to increase the risk for the general population. Poor educational attainment appears to increase risk, but this relationship may equally be explained by other factors such as social class, nutrition, and delayed detection in the 'well-educated'.

Smoking appears to be protective.

At present, the disease is thought to arise from a combination of multifactorial genetic risk factors and, as yet, uncertain environmental factors. Abnormal amyloid deposition appears to be the central pathological process (Fig. 17.2).

Vascular dementia

As with Alzheimer's disease, vascular dementia is closely associated with increasing age. In rare cases, the disease is linked to a dominant gene on chromosone 19 (cerebral autosomal dominant arteriopathy).

The remaining risk factors relate to cerebrovascular disease in general, i.e.:

- Previous stroke.
- Hypertension.
- Diabetes.
- History of myocardial infarct.

Diagnostic criteria for dementia

Core area of deficits/symptoms for dementia are:

- memory
- language
- praxis
- higher intellectual function
- personality and behaviour
- psychosis
- personal functioning
- motor and sensory functioning

At least 6 months of acquired global impairment of intellect, memory and personality is needed. There is no impairment of consciousness and the course is usually chronic and progressive

Fig. 17.1 Diagnostic criteria for dementia.

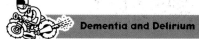

- Carotid artery stenosis.
- Valvular disease.
- Hypercholesterolaemia.
- Hypercoagulation disorders.
- Smoking.
- Male.

Although often termed 'multi-infarct dementia', it is important to remember that dementia can arise from a single infarct.

Diffuse Lewy body dementia

Little is known about the cause of diffuse Lewy body dementia. Allelic variation on the apolipoprotein E gene of chromosome 19 may be linked.

Huntington's disease

Huntington's disease has autosomal dominant inheritance with complete penetrance. It is caused by a variable number triple repeat on the short arm of chromosome 4.

Pick's disease

In familial cases, this disease is linked to an autosomal dominant gene.

Creutzfeldt–Jakob and other prion diseases

The typical pathology of CJD, described in Chapter 6, results from abnormal deposition of the prion (proteinaceous particle) protein in the form of amyloid ß-pleated sheets. Most case are sporadic and of unknown aetiology. Specific causes are:

- Genetic—Gerstmann–Straussler disease, an autosomal dominant condition caused by mutation of PrP gene on chromosome 20.
- Iatrogenic—through inoculation of prions via cadaver growth hormone (prior to genetically engineered products), corneal transplants, stereotactic neurosurgery.
- Consumption of infected food—a famous example is kuru, described in the Fore tribe of Papua New Guinea, a spongiform encephalopathy resulting from cannibalism of neural tissue.

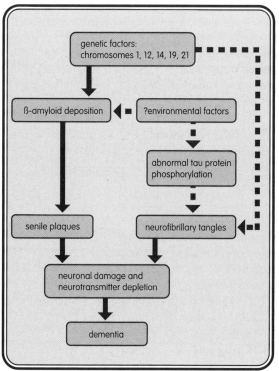

Recently, attention has shifted to consumption of BSE-infected beef products. A link has been postulated with the 'new variant CJD' described recently. It has a younger age of onset, often presents with psychological symptoms, and shows atypical pathological features.

Fig. 17.2 Amyloid cascade theory.

Epidemiology

The overall prevalence of dementia is approximately 0.3% of the total UK population, but it rises sharply with increasing age (Fig. 17. 3): the prevalence in persons aged 45–64 years is approximately 0.035%, whereas that in persons aged 65 or over is approximately 5%.

The relative proportions are:

- Alzheimer's disease, approximately 30–60% cases.
- Vascular dementia, approximately 10–30%.
- Combined Alzheimer's and vascular dementia, approximately 10–30%.
- Lewy body disease, approximately 15%.
- Other causes, less than 5%.

Other epidemiological factors for the main causes of dementia are shown in Fig. 17.4.

Physical and psychological investigations

Physical examination

The main aim of a general physical examination is to identify treatable underlying causes of dementia, such as hypothyroidism or a space-occupying lesion. In addition, consideration should be given to complications of dementia, such as malnutrition or falls.

Cardiovascular and neurological examination are particularly important: evidence of hypertension or circulatory disease has obvious implications for the likelihood of vascular dementia, and neurological examination may identify focal signs necessitating further investigation.

Physical investigations

Apart from HIV-testing for AIDS-associated dementia and genetic tests for Huntington's disease, there are no specific tests for the main forms of dementia described. A list of important screening tests to help diagnose the general medical causes of dementia may be found in Fig. 17.5.

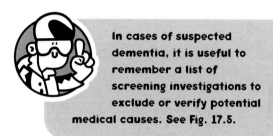

In cases of suspected dementia, it is useful to remember a list of screening investigations to exclude or verify potential medical causes. See Fig. 17.5.

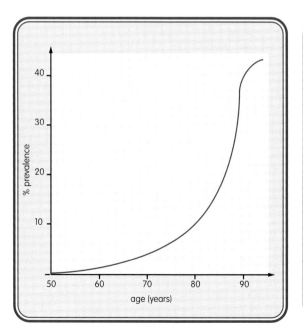

Fig. 17.3 Graph showing increasing prevalence of dementia with age.

Other epidemiological factors for main causes of dementia	
Dementia	**Comments**
Alzheimer's disease	mean age of onset 73 female>male
vascular dementia	male>female
Lewy body dementia	male~female
Huntington's disease	age of onset 25–50 years but 10% >55 years and 10% <20 years male~female; prevalence 4–7/100 000
Pick's disease	female>male age of onset 50–60 years
Creutzfeldt–Jacob disease	female>male 20–50 new cases per year in UK age of onset 50+ years (much younger patients recorded with 'new variant' form)

Fig. 17.4 Other epidemiological factors for the main causes of dementia.

The EEG in most forms of dementia reveals diffuse slowing or loss of a rhythm; it is rarely used unless the clinical picture is atypical or the onset is presenile (<65 years). The typical forms of CJD develop characteristic triphasic sharp wave complexes.

Individual units vary in their use of neuroimaging techniques to help diagnose dementia. Computerized tomography (CT) is used most frequently (Fig. 17.6), although it is gradually being superseded by magnetic resonance imaging (MRI) which is particularly good at identifying small cerebral infarcts. Functional imaging, using positron emission tomography (SPET/PET scans) is also increasingly used to measure variables such as regional blood flow in affected parts of the brain.

Psychological investigations

Psychological investigations are useful when investigating atypical (e.g. predominantly frontal lobe signs) or presenile presentations.

The Mini-Mental State Examination (MMSE) discussed in Chapter 6 is a useful screening and monitoring tool; note that the score naturally declines with age, so that the mean score at 90 years is 23/30. A more thorough

and complex instrument for measuring cognitive skills is the CAMCOG (Cambridge Cognitive Score) questionnaire, which incorporates the MMSE. Specific tests of frontal lobe functioning include the Wisconsin Card Sorting Test.

Complications and prognosis

In addition to the direct consequences of a dementia syndrome—cognitive, psychological, and physical—other indirect associations and complications occur:

- Alzheimer's disease pathology is frequently associated with cerebrovascular disease and Lewy body disease (Parkinson's disease and diffuse forms).
- Increased susceptibility to delirium.
- Increased susceptibility to infections (bronchopneumonia is often a terminal event), malnutrition, and accidents.
- A seven times increased risk of suicide for those diagnosed with Huntington's disease. The rate of suicide for other dementias is not increased.

The course of most dementias is progressive and fatal. Successful treatment of medical causes such as

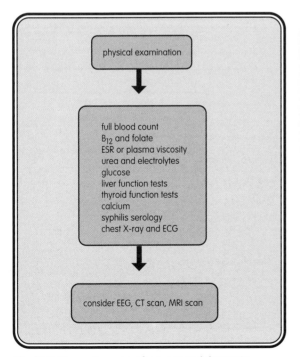

Fig. 17.5 'Dementia screen' for suspected dementia.

Typical CT appearances for main causes of dementia	
Dementia	**CT appearance**
Alzheimer's disease	generalized cerebral atrophy widened sulci dilated ventricles
vascular dementia	cerebral atrophy dilated ventricles single/multiple areas of infarction
Pick's disease	greater relative atrophy of frontal and temporal lobes
Huntington's disease	dilated ventricles atrophy of caudate nuclei
Creutzfeldt–Jacob disease	usually appears normal

Fig. 17.6 Typical CT appearances for the main causes of dementia.

hypothyroidism or hydrocephalus usually arrests rather than resolves the cognitive decline.

Duration of survival from the time of diagnosis for the main causes are shown below:
- Alzheimer's disease—less than 10 years.
- Vascular dementia—variable, given the stepwise fluctuating course.
- Diffuse Lewy body disease—less than 2 years.
- Pick's disease—less than 10 years.
- Huntington's disease—less than 20 years.
- CJD—less than 1 year.

Management

Mention of dementia frequently induces unnecessary hopelessness and therapeutic nihilism among doctors. There is the likelihood of specific pharmacological treatments becoming established, and considerable improvements in a patient's quality of life can be achieved through a variety of approaches.

The principles of management are:
- Treating the underlying cause if possible (e.g. hypothyroidism, modifying vascular risk factors).
- Treating associated disorders or complications (e.g. aggression, chest infections, incontinence).
- Addressing functional problems that result (e.g. kitchen skills, financial management, social isolation).
- Providing advice and support for carers.

Assessment and treatment of these areas can usually be done in a primary care or outpatient setting; occasionally there is a need to admit patients into a dementia-assessment ward or day hospital, particularly when behavioural problems are severe. Dementia often presents on an acute medical ward after treatment of a comorbid delirium, or due to the disorientating effects of the new environment itself.

Specific management strategies
Pharmacological
Disturbed behaviour such as aggression or agitation may be treated with conventional antipsychotics (commonly promazine and haloperidol) or benzodiazepines. Low doses are vital since the elderly may be slow metabolizers and they show greater susceptibility to Parkinsonian side effects. All of these drugs may worsen cognitive function; particularly those with a strong anticholinergic action.

Psychosis and depressive symptoms may be treated with conventional antipsychotics and antidepressants.

Recently, drugs have been introduced to specifically treat Alzheimer's disease. Both tacrine and donepezil increase central cholinergic activity by inhibiting acetylcholinesterase enzymes. Donepezil has recently been licensed for use in the United Kingdom: it appears to slow down the deterioration in cognitive function associated with Alzheimer's disease, although its longer-term role in management is uncertain.

Psychological
Several cognitive–behavioural methods can be employed:
- Behavioural therapy may replace or augment drug treatments in the control of behaviour disturbance.
- Reality orientation makes concerted efforts to inform awareness of time and place, such as prominent clocks or calendars.
- Reminiscence therapy highlights pleasurable but distant memories, which are least affected by dementia.

Finally, it is important to providing genetic counselling for patients undergoing investigation for the Huntington's disease gene.

Treating diffuse Lewy body disease with antipsychotics is often catastrophic, causing severe Parkinsonian symptoms and rapid physical deterioration. Benzodiazepines are safer in this group of patients. This exemplifies the need to exercise caution when prescribing antipsychotics and the need to try to differentiate clinically the types of dementia.

Social

As dementia causes such a profound deterioration in functional abilities, careful evaluation of need is required. The assessments of social workers, occupational therapists, and physiotherapists are all important in this respect.

It is preferable to keep patients in their own environment, as sudden unfamiliarity frequently causes greater distress and disorientation. If the patient lives alone or has severe behavioural or physical disabilities, residential, nursing, or specialist EMI (elderly mental illness) homes need to be considered.

It is important to provide practical advice and support for carers, such as regular respite care for their relation and access to local support groups.

DELIRIUM

The diagnostic criteria for delirium are shown in Fig. 17.7.

Aetiology

An underlying medical or drug-related cause of delirium, as listed in Chapter 6 is usually identified. Exact pathophysiological mechanisms for delirium remain unclear.

Postulated mechanisms include:
- Alterations in cholinergic and noradrenergic neurotransmitter systems.
- Interruption of normal information-processing systems.
- Interruption of the blood–brain barrier.

Epidemiology

Most research into the epidemiology of delirium concentrates on the elderly, who, along with infants and young children, are more vulnerable to this disorder. The prevalence in persons aged over 65 admitted to hospital is approximately 10%. The incidence in the over-65s during hospitalization is 20–30%.

Physical investigations

Similar principles to the investigation of dementia apply to delirium, particularly since there is usually an identifiable organic cause. Additional investigations to consider include C-reactive protein (marker of infection), arterial blood gases, blood and urine cultures, virology, and urine drug screen.

EEG shows diffuse slowing and may be useful if encephalitis is suspected.

Prognosis

The average duration of delirium is 7 days. Inpatients who develop delirium have an increased mortality; this is unsurprising given the often serious nature of the underlying medical conditions. Cognitive dysfunction commonly presents after the delirium has resolved; this may reflect pre-existing dementia or damage secondary to the delirium.

Management

Delirium can be highly distressing for patients and anxiety-provoking for medical ward staff unfamiliar with 'psychiatric problems'.

General principles of management are as follows:
- Try to nurse in a well-lit, quiet environment, preferably a side room.
- Maximize visual acuity and hearing ability to avoid misinterpretation of stimuli.
- Encourage familiar faces to visit and 'orientate' the patient.
- Avoid sedative medication if possible, particularly drugs with a powerful anticholinergic effect such as thioridazine—low-dose haloperidol, trifluoperazine, or benzodiazepines are preferable.
- Vigorously investigate and treat any underlying medical condition.

The specific management of delirium tremens is outlined in Chapter 18.

Diagnostic criteria for delirium

An acute/subacute syndrome characterized by fluctuating disturbances in consciousness accompanied by changes in:
- cognition (memory, judgement, orientation, thinking, perception)
- psychomotor function
- sleep–wake cycle
- affect

Fig. 17.7 Diagnostic criteria for delirium.

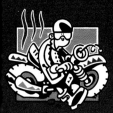

18. Alcohol and Substance Misuse

The classification of substance misuse disorders is summarized in Fig. 18.1.

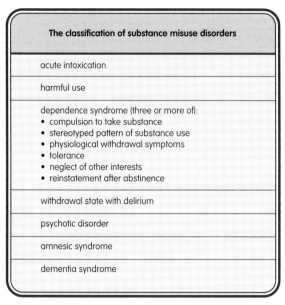

The classification of substance misuse disorders
acute intoxication
harmful use
dependence syndrome (three or more of): • compulsion to take substance • stereotyped pattern of substance use • physiological withdrawal symptoms • tolerance • neglect of other interests • reinstatement after abstinence
withdrawal state with delirium
psychotic disorder
amnesic syndrome
dementia syndrome

Fig. 18.1 The classification of substance misuse disorders.

ALCOHOL AND SUBSTANCE DEPENDENCE

Aetiology
Most of the discussion in this section will relate to the aetiological factors associated with alcohol dependence although there is overlap with other forms of substance misuse.

It is now widely accepted that the causes of alcohol dependence are multifactorial and encompass a 'biopsychosocial' approach, in common with many other psychiatric disorders.

Biological theories
Genetic predisposition
Most family studies show an increased risk of dependence among relatives of dependent individuals; adoption studies indicate a heritable component, as offspring of dependent parents have higher rates of dependence than their non-dependent adoptive parents. The nature of this influence is unclear. It may operate at the level of heritable personality characteristics or it might relate to the body's biochemical susceptibility to alcohol and its consequences. For example, 50% of east-Asian populations have a deficiency in one of the aldehyde dehydrogenase enzymes, leading to flushing and palpitations after small quantities of alcohol—this may explain reduced rates of consumption and dependence in these cultures.

Biochemical
The biochemical basis of dependence remains uncertain. A current model postulates decreasing activity of GABA-ergic systems and increasing activity of glutamate systems in response to chronic alcohol administration. The former is facilitated by increasing calcium channels which reduce chloride ion flow. By decreasing the inhibitory actions of GABA to counteract the CNS depressant effects of alcohol, the neurons become more excitable and this leads to the symptoms of CNS excitability that occur on sudden alcohol withdrawal.

Psychological theories
Psychodynamic
Several theories have been developed by the various schools of psychoanalytic thinking. One theory suggests there are unconscious gains resulting from both intoxication (allows release of aggression) and the personal damage caused (sympathy from others).

Cognitive–behavioural
Cognitive–behavioural theories are based on associative learning (classical and operant conditioning), cognitive learning, and social learning theories. In the associative learning theory, a neutral (unconditioned) stimulus such as a pub becomes associated with alcohol; this then becomes a

conditioned stimulus, leading to psychological craving. An alternative explanation, according to social learning theory, is that patterns of alcohol consumption are modelled on the drinking behaviour of relatives or peers. Family studies support the idea that drinking habits follow those of older relatives.

Personality factors

There is little evidence to support the notion of an underlying 'addictive personality', although there is evidence linking dependence with premorbid dissocial and borderline personality traits.

Psychiatric disorders

Psychotic, affective, and anxiety disorders appear to increase the risk of alcohol dependence.

Social and environmental theories

Levels of alcohol consumption

Population levels of alcohol consumption are closely related to levels of alcohol-related disorders which in turn are related to the easily measurable number of deaths from cirrhosis. There are wide variations among populations in this respect, e.g. levels in Italy and France are greater than those in the UK and USA. Levels of consumption are influenced by the real cost of alcohol (in relation to incomes) and availability. Other cultural factors such as attitudes to heavy drinking interact to increase national differences.

Occupation

There is a clear link between certain occupations and deaths from cirrhosis; again, issues of availability and subcultural attitudes interplay. The highest-risk professions are members of leisure and catering trades (publicans especially), and those involved with shipping and travel. However, when one looks at the overall picture, higher rates of dependence are noted in unskilled workers and the unemployed, compared to the higher social classes; this may be partly explained by the 'social drift' caused by alcohol dependence (see Chapter 19).

Significant life events

Significant life events appear to increase the amounts of alcohol consumed and therefore the risk of dependence.

Illicit-drug dependence

The aetiological factors for illicit-drug dependence are even less well understood, although would again appear to be related to a mixture of biopsychosocial factors. Factors of price, availability, and cultural attitudes again appear to operate at a population level. Moreover, social deprivation, a family environment of substance misusers, conduct disorder in childhood, dissocial personality disorder, and severe mental illness increase the likelihood of substance-misuse problems.

The introduction of harsher legal penalties for suppliers and users of illicit drugs, and increased education about the effects of drug use, have not resulted in a decrease in illicit-drug use over the last 30 years.

Epidemiology

Accurate figures are difficult to obtain given the complexities of assessing what is still stigmatized and socially undesirable behaviour. Estimates are based on population surveys, hospital-admission statistics, and cirrhosis statistics (for alcohol).

Alcohol

Prevalence

Ten per cent of the UK adult population are completely abstinent.

Figures based on general-practice surveys are as follows:
- Risky drinking without problems—7% female, 3% male.
- Harmful use, no dependence—2% female, 7% male.
- Alcohol dependence—2% female, 7% male.

USA figures for alcohol dependence (based on a structured diagnostic questionnaire) are:
- Lifetime prevalence—14%.
- Prevalence in last year—7%.

Demography

Alcohol can be characterized demographically as follows:
- Marital status—divorced/separated>single>married.
- Age—the highest consumption of alcohol occurs for both sexes in the age band 18–24 years, but problems related to dependence tend to emerge at a later age.

- Social class—as has been mentioned above, alcohol consumption is higher in social class V and the unemployed. This picture applies particularly to men. In women, higher rates of consumption are seen in the higher social classes.

Illicit substances
Prevalence
As with alcohol, overall illicit-substance use has increased over the last 30 years. Rates are particularly high within urban, socially deprived areas.
Figures are as follows:
- 20–30% of people aged 16–59 years have taken an illegal substance.
- 50% of people aged 16–29 years have taken an illegal substance.
- 18% of people aged 16–29 years have taken an illegal substance in the last month (of whom 3% are injecting); 5% in this age group have taken two or more illegal substances in the last month.

Type of drug used
In general, cannabis is most commonly used, followed by amphetamine, ecstasy, and LSD; heroin is used less frequently, and cocaine has not reached the same proportions of use in the UK as it has in the USA.

Sex differences
Using the Home Office Addicts Index 1991, the male:female ratio of the 20 000 listed is 3:1.

Investigations
Physical examination
The physical examination is an important part of any assessment of substance-use problems and requires an awareness of the acute and long-term effects of substance use.
The following areas should be considered:
- Evidence of acute use or intoxication, e.g. pupillary constriction associated with opiate use.
- Immediate and short-term medical complications of substance use, e.g. head injury following alcohol intoxication, local infection and abscesses caused by intravenous substance use.
- Signs of substance withdrawal, e.g. raised blood pressure, tachycardia, sweating, and pupil dilatation, associated with alcohol or benzodiazepine withdrawal.

- Long-term medical complications, e.g. stigmata of liver disease associated with alcohol (or infectious hepatitis caused by intravenous drug use).

Physical investigations
General
A wide range of non-specific investigations can be useful when the longer-term medical complications of substance misuse are suspected: these include full blood count (FBC), urea and electrolytes (U/Es), liver function tests (LFTs), ECG, chest x-ray (CXR), hepatitis serology, and an HIV test. If the patient is suffering withdrawal with delirium, additional investigations looking for other complicating causes (particularly infection) are required, e.g. erythrocyte sedimentation rate (ESR), C-reactive protein (CRP), blood cultures.

Specific
Specific investigations for evidence of excessive alcohol consumption include:
- ↑Mean corpuscular volume (MCV)—this occurs in 60%, females more than males, and is due to a deficiency of vitamin B or as a direct effect on erythropoiesis.
- ↑Gamma-glutamyl transpeptidase (γ-GT)—this occurs in 80%; other liver function tests are usually increased once there is advanced liver disease.
- Blood alcohol or a breathalyzer detects recent use (it takes 24 hours to be fully excreted).
- ↑Serum carbohydrate-deficient transferrin detects excessive use (>7 units/day) in the previous 7 days.
- ↑Triglycerides and ↑cholesterol.
- ↑White cell count (WCC), ↑ESR, and ↑LFTs—these occur in delirium tremens.

Illicit-substance use
Urine drug screens are listed in Fig. 18.2.

A urine drug screen should be considered for all psychiatric admissions; particularly young, psychotic patients. Because the half-lives of some of the drugs are short, collect the urine as soon as possible.

Fig. 18.2 Urine drug screens.

Urine drug screens		
Drug	**Length of time detectable in urine**	**Comments**
opiates	12–36 hours several days	short acting long acting
amphetamine	1–3 days	—
cocaine	1–3 days 7–12 days	— repeated high doses
benzodiazepines	7 days	longer acting substances
cannabis	7–10 days 2–4 weeks	— heavy use
phencyclidine	several weeks	repeated high doses

Complications

Medical

Alcohol dependence, in particular, gives rise to significant morbidity and reduction in life expectancy. This derives from both direct and indirect effects.

Ten per cent of alcohol-dependent patients develop cirrhosis; females are more susceptible than males. The 5-year mortality figures are 10% if abstinence achieved, 40% if drinking continues, and 65% in advanced disease.

Indirect effects of alcohol include increased accidents, obesity (or malnutrition), and neglect of other conditions (e.g. diabetes).

Overall mortality rate is twice the expected. Excessive alcohol consumption is reported in 10–20% of general medical admissions. Drinkers who remain within safe drinking limits appear to have a lower mortality than lifelong abstainers; this may be related to a cardioprotective effect of alcohol.

Morbidity associated with illicit-substance misuse particularly affects injecting drug users. One London and South East study found rates of HIV infection at 3–4%.

Psychological

The close association between substance misuse and psychotic, affective, and anxiety disorders was highlighted in Chapter 7; lifetime risks of suicide for both alcohol and illicit-drug dependence are around 10%.

Social

The social cost of alcohol can be measured in several ways:

- Drink driving—even at the legal limit (80 mg/100 ml), inexperienced drivers are at a five times higher risk of an accident, and a third of all killed drivers are above the legal limit.
- Violent crime—in up to 50% of murders, one of the participants is intoxicated, and up to 70% of violent crime is near licensed premises.

A similar pattern of social consequences occurs with illicit-substance misuse, particularly acquisitive crime (shoplifting, burglary, etc.)—up to 30% of thefts from the person are committed by the drug-dependent.

Management

The principles of management are similar for both alcohol and substance dependence:

- Short-term—treating the acute effects of the substance, such as intoxication or withdrawal syndromes.
- Medium-term—rehabilitating patient after withdrawal.
- Long-term—dealing with the medical, psychological, and social consequences listed above.

Good prognostic indicators for patients are:

- In a stable relationship.
- Employed.

- Stable living conditions with good social supports.
- Good insight into problems and self-motivation to change.

Service provision for this group of patients is diverse; most districts employ either a specialist addictions psychiatrist or a general adult psychiatrist with an interest in substance misuse. In addition, Community Psychiatric Nurses (CPNs) may develop a specialist interest in this area, and work in association with local and national voluntary organizations. Emphasis is placed on multidisciplinary management and harm-reduction.

Alcohol

As with all disorders, it is important to consider medical, psychological, and social dimensions to management.

Medical

Detoxification The management of alcohol withdrawal is shown in Fig. 18.3.

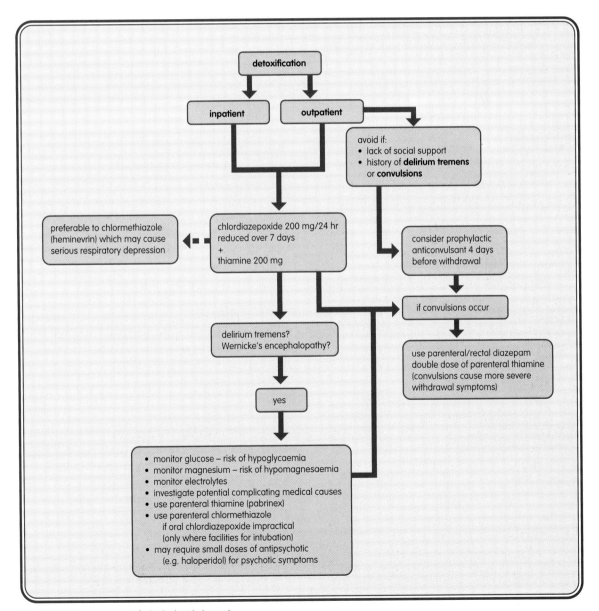

Fig. 18.3 Management of alcohol withdrawal.

Alcohol withdrawal is highly unpleasant for the patient and can have serious medical consequences if not carefully managed. Untreated delirium tremens has a mortality rate of around 5%.

Learn the clinical features and management of alcohol withdrawal thoroughly; it commonly arises unexpectedly on both medical and surgical wards.

Associated psychiatric conditions Alcohol hallucinosis may be treated with standard antipsychotics. Caution must be exercised when prescribing antidepressants to the alcohol-dependent owing to the risk of intentional or non-intentional overdose; older tricyclics should be avoided.

Maintenance after detoxification

- Disulfiram (Antabuse)—blocks alcohol oxidation, leading to accumulation of acetaldehyde. This causes unpleasant symptoms of anxiety, flushing, palpitations, headache, and a choking sensation within 20 minutes of alcohol consumption. The drug is usually taken orally, although surgical implants are available. Rarely, it causes death through arrhythmias, therefore baseline cardiovascular investigations are advised.
- Acamprosate (Campral)—enhances GABA transmission and appears to reduce the likelihood of relapse after detoxification. It is a relatively new drug and its long-term role has yet to be determined.
- Benzodiazepines—continuing use after detoxification is controversial because of their own dependence potential and cumulative CNS depressant effect. Ideally, they should be avoided.

Note, use of any maintenance treatment requires careful supervision and continued psychosocial intervention.

Psychological and social

Supportive psychotherapy Early recognition, advice, and explanation of alcohol problems is a particularly effective intervention which does not need specialist training. Alcohol-dependent patients may benefit from further supportive counselling, both before and after detoxification; this may be done in individual or group settings (e.g. Alcoholics Anonymous).

Cognitive–behavioural psychotherapy This has been shown to help patients avoid relapse after detoxification. It might include, for example, learning strategies to avoid 'high-risk situations' such as walking past a pub.

Social As indicated above, best results are achieved against a background of social stability; it is important to consider issues such as relationship problems, debt, homelessness, and criminal charges in any management plan. Other professionals such as social workers and probation officers may have an important role in this area. Support and advice for carers is particularly important.

Primary prevention Increasing the real cost of alcohol appears to be the most effective strategy in reducing overall consumption in the whole population. Changing availability, advertising, or encouraging health education appears to have little effect.

Illicit substances

The principles applied to the management of illicit substances are the same as those used for alcohol dependence; specific features of management for each will be discussed below.

Opiates

Maintenance treatment of opiate use can be offered by converting patients to the longer-acting oral opioid methadone. It helps break the cycle of regular use and prevents the complications of injecting. Before prescribing, opiate use should be proven by a urine drug screen—serious respiratory depression may result if the patient is not already tolerant to opiates.

Detoxification can be facilitated by gradual reduction in methadone over the course of a few days. Withdrawal is distressing although not life threatening.

The symptoms may be ameliorated by lofexidine (a centrally acting α-adrenoceptor agonist), loperamide (for diarrhoea), buscopan (for stomach cramps), and hyoscine (for nausea).

Once detoxified, naltrexone (an opiate antagonist) is sometimes used to block the euphoriant effects of any continued opiate use. It induces withdrawal if the patient is still dependent.

Benzodiazepines

As with alcohol, caution must be exercised when attempting a managed withdrawal from benzodiazepines. Patients are initially converted from short-acting (e.g. lorazepam, temazepam) to long-acting compounds (usually diazepam). Doses are then reduced very slowly, e.g. by an eighth of the dose every week.

Cocaine and amphetamine

Both cocaine and amphetamine can be stopped abruptly. Antidepressants may help the depressed mood that follows withdrawal from heavy use.

Psychotic disorders induced by these drugs benefit from symptomatic treatment with short courses of benzodiazepines or antipsychotics.

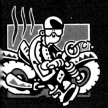

19. Psychotic Disorders

Among the psychotic disorders, the main ones that should be distinguished are schizophrenia, delusional disorders, acute and transient psychoses, and schizoaffective disorders. This chapter will concentrate on schizophrenia, the most important and widely researched disorder in this group.

SCHIZOPHRENIA

Historical aspects

Ideas about the disorder we now term schizophrenia crystallized towards the end of the last century. The concept of this disorder has evolved during this century. Important landmarks in the definition of this disorder are:

- 1893—Emil Kraepelin separated affective psychoses (e.g. mania) from non-affective psychoses; he gave the term 'dementia praecox' to clinical conditions resembling the main forms of schizophrenia.
- 1911—Eugen Bleuler coined the term 'schizophrenia' ('splitting of psychic functions'); his description placed more emphasis on thought-disorder and negative symptoms than on positive symptoms.
- 1959—Kurt Schneider defined first-rank symptoms, which now comprise the first three sets of criteria for the ICD-10 definition (Fig. 19.1).
- 1970–present—international classification systems have further clarified the diagnostic criteria; the main distinction between ICD-10 and DSM-IV is that the latter specifies a 6-month duration of symptoms and places more emphasis on social or occupational dysfunction.

Aetiological theories

Schizophrenia appears to be secondary to a complex interaction of biological and environmental factors. Important elements of this biopsychosocial model will be described in turn.

Genetic

There is a strong tendency for schizophrenia to run in families (Fig. 19.2).

Evaluation of adoption studies provides further supporting evidence for a genetic factor: babies

---

Diagnostic criteria for schizophrenia

A) One (or more) symptom from any of these groups:

- thought echo, thought insertion/withdrawal/broadcasting
- delusions of control, delusional perception
- auditory hallucinations in the third person, running commentary form or from another part of the body
- persistent completely impossible delusions

B) Two (or more) symptoms from any of these groups:

- persistent hallucinations in any modality +/– delusions/ overvalued ideas
- thought disorder
- catatonia
- negative symptoms

One month or more of the A symptoms and/or of the B symptoms

Fig. 19.1 Diagnostic criteria for schizophrenia.

Lifetime risk of schizophrenia for relatives of schizophrenic patients

Relation	Percentage schizophrenic
monozygotic twin	50
both parents	50
parent and one sibling	17
sibling or dizygotic twin	10
one parent	6
grandparent	4
uncles, aunts, nieces, nephews	3
general population	<1

Fig. 19.2 Lifetime risk of schizophrenia for relatives of schizophrenic patients.

adopted away from schizophrenic parents to non-schizophrenic parents retain their increased risk, whereas the risk is not increased when babies are adopted to schizophrenic parents from non-schizophrenic biological parents.

The mechanism for this inheritance is unknown although several candidate genes are emerging. As concordance is well below 100% for even monozygotic twins, genetics can only provide part of the story.

Developmental factors

Strong evidence is now emerging that schizophrenia is associated with complications during pregnancy and birth. In addition, the observation that more schizophrenics are born in late winter or spring has led to the theory that schizophrenia is linked to second-trimester influenza infection.

Brain abnormalities

Increasingly sophisticated neuroimaging techniques are starting to consistently identify structural and functional abnormalities associated with schizophrenia; the findings may be secondary to the disorder itself or its treatment. They include:

- Ventricular enlargement (appears to be associated with negative symptoms).
- Generalized reduction in brain volume.
- Abnormalities of frontal and temporal lobes—particularly left sided.

Furthermore, schizophrenics have been found to perform worse at specific tests of frontal lobe function and demonstrate 'soft' neurological signs, e.g. abnormalities of stereognosis or proprioception.

Neurotransmitter abnormalities

Based largely on the effects of antipsychotic drugs, the dopamine theory suggests that schizophrenia is secondary to overactivity of dopamine pathways between the midbrain, cerebral cortex, and limbic system (mesocortical and mesolimbic pathways). Drugs that potentiate these pathways such as amphetamine or antiparkinsonian agents are known to cause psychosis. The recent identification of several dopamine receptor subtypes and successful use of clozapine (which blocks both dopamine and serotonin receptors) suggests a more complex mechanism than previously thought.

Life events

Stressful life events occur more frequently in the month before a first psychotic episode or relapse, and may therefore precipitate the illness. This finding could alternatively be explained by the early stages of the illness itself causing the events.

Expressed emotion

When family or carers become over-involved, over-critical, or hostile towards a schizophrenic patient, he or she is more likely to relapse. This interaction has been termed 'high expressed emotion' and only exerts an influence if contact is greater than 35 hours a week.

Epidemiology

Details of the epidemiology of schizophrenia are given in Fig. 19.3.

Investigations

In patients presenting with a psychosis, further investigations are necessary to:

- Exclude an organic cause for the disorder.
- Exclude comorbid physical disease.
- Take baseline physical measures before treatment.

There are no diagnostic tests for schizophrenia and its related disorders; the neuropsychological and brain abnormalities described earlier are based on comparisons between groups of patients and controls—they are too subtle to use clinically.

A basic physical examination will usually suffice for a patient admitted with a relapse of a known psychotic disorder.

If the patient presents with a first episode of psychosis, it is usual to augment the examination with investigations: a good basic screen comprises full blood count (FBC), erythrocyte sedimentation rate (ESR), urea and electrolytes (U/Es), thyroid function, liver function tests (LFT), glucose, and serum calcium. The additional investigations of a 'dementia screen' are worthwhile in elderly patients. The use of a routine EEG or CT scan to help exclude an organic psychosis varies between units; they should always be considered in atypical cases, cases with treatment resistance, or if there are cognitive abnormalities.

A urine drug screen should always be done because illicit drugs both cause and exacerbate a psychosis.

Epidemiology of schizophrenia	
Variable	**Comments**
prevalence and incidence	point prevalence: 0.3–0.6/100 lifetime risk: 0.7–0.9/100, i.e. almost 1% incidence: 0.02–0.04/100 per year
sex distribution	males~females
age of onset	peak for males: 15–25 peak for females: 25–35 episodes can begin at any age, although are rare in childhood and early adolescence
social class	rates are higher in lower social classes, this has been attributed to social drift, i.e. the deterioration in personal functioning secondary to the disorder results in movement down the social scale
geography	rates are higher in urban compared to rural areas, again this may be accounted by social drift overall rates are remarkably similar across different countries even where cultures differ, e.g. India and UK
migration	several studies have shown increased rates in migrant populations, e.g. Afro-Caribbean immigrants to the UK. In this example, rates are even higher in the second generation; this may reflect socio-economic deprivation, racism, increased illicit substance use, or diagnostic bias amongst clinicians

Fig. 19.3 Epidemiology of schizophrenia.

Course and prognosis

Course

The course of schizophrenia is highly variable and difficult to predict for individual patients. In general, the disorder is chronic, showing a relapsing and remitting pattern; the type of symptoms are usually similar for each relapse, although they decrease in severity over time.

The following patterns emerge:
- Single lifetime episode—approximately 20%.
- Repeated episodes with return to normal functioning in-between—approximately 35%.
- Repeated episodes without return to normal functioning in-between—approximately 10%.
- Repeated episodes with progressive impairment of personal functioning in-between—approximately 35%.

The influence of modern drug treatments and deinstitutionalization on long-term prognosis have yet to be fully evaluated.

The lifespan for schizophrenic patients is on average 10 years shorter than for the general population; much of this is due to the approximate 10% lifetime risk of suicide. Indirect factors include increased smoking, socioeconomic deprivation, neglect of diet, and accidents.

Those at most risk of suicide are typically young, intelligent males with persistent delusions and hallucinations but good or partial insight.

Prognosis

The overall prognosis for schizophrenia appears to be better in developing as opposed to developed countries; the reasons are unclear but may reflect better extended-family social support or greater social acceptance once recovered. Nevertheless, in the developed world, most patients return to normal or near-normal personal functioning after psychotic episodes and only a small minority require full time care or supervision.

The factors associated with a good prognosis are listed in Fig. 19.4; poor prognostic factors are the converse of these.

Good prognostic factors for schizophrenia
female older age of onset married good premorbid personal and social functioning absence of previous psychiatric history acute onset short episode onset precipitated by life stress good response to medication

Fig. 19.4 Good prognostic factors for schizophrenia.

Management

Patients presenting with an acute psychosis have a variety of needs and the individual management plan must be tailored accordingly.

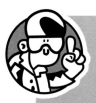

It is useful to divide management according to short-term, medium-term, and long-term factors; considering medical, psychological, and social approaches for each.

Medical treatment

Antipsychotics

Antipsychotics, a diverse category of drugs, have formed the mainstay of treatment for psychoses since the 1950s. They relieve distress and help to control behaviour disturbance (Fig. 19.5). Their antipsychotic action (relieving positive symptoms—delusions and hallucinations) is delayed for about 2 weeks after initiation. Approximately 75% of patients respond to conventional antipsychotics although these have little effect on negative symptoms. Maintenance treatment reduces the risk of relapse.

A drug-free assessment (of about 1 week) should be considered if the onset of psychosis was acute (<1 month) and the diagnosis is unclear. However, patients are more likely to respond if treatment is initiated early. When the diagnosis is already established, or the symptoms are chronic and distressing; it is best to initiate antipsychotic treatment.

As antipsychotics have equivalent efficacy (clozapine excepted), the choice of drug should be guided by previous knowledge of a patient's response to antipsychotics and their susceptibility to side effects such as hypotension and dystonia. If the patient has never been treated with antipsychotics, clinicians tend to choose drugs they are familiar with.

Starting doses should be small to minimize adverse reactions and then increased according to clinical response. As the antipsychotic effect is delayed, this should ideally be done at no shorter than 2-weekly intervals.

The length of treatment requires careful consideration as single episodes cannot be predicted and most patients with schizophrenia relapse. After a first episode, treatment may be gradually stopped after 6–8 months; for most patients, antipsychotics are a long-term, perhaps lifelong, treatment. Depot preparations may be considered to improve long-term compliance.

If the patient fails to respond to a conventional antipsychotic or develops intolerable side effects, an alternative is usually tried using the same procedures as above. In practice the new atypicals, e.g. olanzapine or risperidone, are tried as second or third line drugs. If a patient is 'treatment resistant' to two or more antipsychotics, clozapine is considered—this drug benefits up to 60% of treatment-resistant patients as well as benefiting negative symptoms.

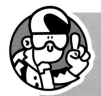

Note that injections given under Common Law should only be used once; if repeat injections are necessary, consider use of the Mental Health Act. Always carefully monitor pulse, blood pressure (examine fully when patient is amenable); try to establish on regular oral or depot medication as soon as possible.

Benzodiazepines

Benzodiazepines can be of enormous benefit in short-term relief of behaviour disturbance, insomnia, and agitation, but do not have any specific antipsychotic effect.

Antidepressants and lithium

Antidepressants and lithium can be used to augment antipsychotics when there are significant affective symptoms, as is the case in schizoaffective disorders, or post schizophrenia depression.

ECT

ECT is now rarely used in schizophrenia, particularly as treatment-resistant patients are now offered clozapine.

The usual indication are the rare cases with severe catatonic symptoms.

Acute behaviour disturbance

Severe disturbance as a result of psychomotor agitation or aggressive behaviour frequently occurs in acutely ill psychotic patients. The algorithm in Fig. 19.5 illustrates the principles of acute management.

Psychological treatments

Until recently, psychotic disorders were thought to be unresponsive to psychological interventions, but increasing evidence points towards their value in augmenting drug treatments.

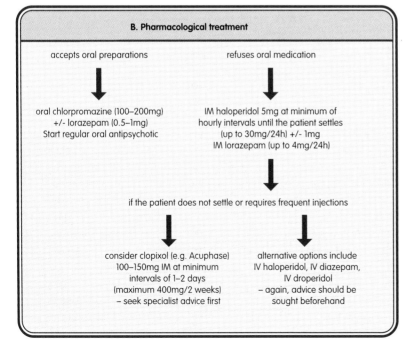

A. Environmental factors

- assess the patient in a quiet environment where external stimulation is kept to a minimum
- ensure safety of yourself and other staff (no heroics!):
  place yourself between the patient and the door to aid escape
  ensure other staff are at hand, preferably with control and restraint training
  don't assess alone if you feel threatened
- try to gain the trust of the patient, avoiding confrontation
- if giving medication against the patient's will (e.g. under common law), explain why you are taking this course of action; document reasons carefully in the notes – try voluntary treatment first

B. Pharmacological treatment

accepts oral preparations

oral chlorpromazine (100–200mg)
+/- lorazepam (0.5–1mg)
Start regular oral antipsychotic

refuses oral medication

IM haloperidol 5mg at minimum of hourly intervals until the patient settles (up to 30mg/24h) +/- 1mg IM lorazepam (up to 4mg/24h)

if the patient does not settle or requires frequent injections

consider clopixol (e.g. Acuphase) 100–150mg IM at minimum intervals of 1–2 days (maximum 400mg/2 weeks) – seek specialist advice first

alternative options include IV haloperidol, IV diazepam, IV droperidol – again, advice should be sought beforehand

Fig. 19.5 Management of acute behaviour disturbance. A. Environmental factors and B. Pharmacological treatment.

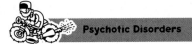

The disorder is often highly distressing, patients frequently lack insight into their illness, and treatments have unpleasant side effects; therefore it is important to provide support, advice, reassurance, and education to both patients and carers in order to build trust and confidence into their management.

Specific family interventions are designed to reduce the effects of high expressed emotions among carers.

Cognitive–behavioural techniques may be used to challenge persistent delusions, relieve persistent hallucinations, and improve treatment compliance. Social-skills training can help longer-term rehabilitation.

Psychoanalysis is usually contraindicated during psychotic illnesses but is sometimes used after psychotic symptoms have resolved.

Social aspects of management

Issues beyond drug and psychological treatment should be addressed to enable successful rehabilitation into the community; these include financial benefits, occupation, accommodation, daytime activities, social supports, and support for carers. A variety of agencies can provide these services; notably, health services, social services, local authorities, local support groups, and national support groups (NSF, SANE, MIND).

All patients with schizophrenia should be assessed for the care-programme approach (CPA) to achieve optimum coordination in the delivery of services. Community psychiatric nurses or social workers are often the appointed keyworkers.

20. Affective Disorders

This chapter includes:

- Depressive disorders.
- Bipolar affective disorder.
- Cyclothymia.
- Dysthymia.

Diagnosis of these conditions has been discussed in Chapter 1.

DEPRESSIVE DISORDERS

Aetiology

Biological and genetic factors

It has long been thought that depression may have a biological basis. Monoamine theories of depression suggest that the illness is linked to a lack of availability of noradrenaline, serotonin, and possibly dopamine. These monoamines influence second-messenger systems to alter production of intracellular proteins.

One strength of the monoamine theory is that the actions of antidepressants can easily be conceptualized in the framework it provides. Tricyclic drugs primarily prevent noradrenaline reuptake, making more available in the synaptic cleft. Selective serotonin reuptake inhibitors (SSRIs) have a similar action and increase serotonin levels. Monoamine oxidase inhibitors (MAOIs) prevent noradrenaline breakdown presynaptically, so that more is available for release. Each class of drug makes more monoamine molecules available in the synaptic cleft; these monoamines act postsynaptically, reactivating the second messengers, which, over time, may reverse intracellular changes and provide a remission of symptoms.

It is likely that the monoamine theory is an oversimplification and that transmitter substances such as GABA and peptides (e.g. vasopressin) are also involved. It has been suggested that depressive disorders may be linked to abnormalities in the regulation of corticosteroids through disturbances in the hypothalamic–pituitary–adrenal axis, or to disturbances in the lipid constituents of neuronal membranes.

Twin and family studies have shown that there is a genetic basis to many cases of depression; hence, a family history in a first-degree relative is a significant risk factor for depressive disorders.

Psychological and social factors

There is strong evidence that psychological factors (e.g. maternal deprivation or other childhood loss) may predispose to depression. Depression is known to be associated with hysterical and obsessive–compulsive (anankastic) personalities and with significant adverse life events such as marital separation and job loss. Other social risk factors include being at home with young children, having no external employment, and lacking close confidant(e)s.

Epidemiology

Depression is common, with up to 18% of the population experiencing a depressive episode at some point in their lives. Females are at greater risk than males by a ratio of 2:1. A first depressive episode may occur at any age, the mean onset being in the late 30s, with peaks at 30 years and 50 years.

Investigations

Investigations for patients with suspected depressive disorders are usually performed to rule out organic causes. Such investigations include:

- Full blood count—check for anaemia, infection (raised white count), and a high mean cell volume (MCV; a marker of alcoholism).
- Urea and electrolytes—check for renal problems.
- Liver function tests.
- Thyroid function tests and calcium.
- Vitamin B_{12} and folate.
- Urine drug screen.
- Sometimes, a VDRL test—check for syphilis.

Despite much research on the dexamethasone suppression test (DST), there is no reliable blood test to indicate the presence of depression. However, one biological finding that is strongly associated with depression is a reduction in the latency (time to onset after falling asleep) of rapid eye movement (REM) sleep.

153

Course and prognosis

Depression is self-limiting, and without treatment a first depressive episode will generally remit within 6 months to 1 year. However, the course of depression is often chronic and relapsing, leading to a diagnosis of recurrent depressive disorder.

Good prognostic features in depression include:
- Lesser severity of episode (mild better than moderate, moderate better than severe).
- Absence of psychotic features.
- Absence of comorbid psychiatric illness (including personality disorders and alcohol or substance abuse).
- Existence of confidant(e)s.

Depression is one of the most important risk factors for suicide, with age-adjusted rates of suicide being over 20 times greater among patients with major depression compared with those in the general population.

Management setting

Most patients with depression can be treated successfully in primary care or else in psychiatric outpatients. Day-hospital attendance may be helpful in patients with chronic or recurrent illness, especially if poor motivation or low self-esteem has led to a reluctance to go outside the home and make contact with others. Inpatient admission may be advisable for assessment of patients with:
- Bizarre or distressing hallucinations or other psychotic phenomena.
- Active suicidal ideation or planning, especially if suicide has previously been attempted or many risk factors for suicide are present.
- Other deliberate self-harm.
- Lack of motivation leading to self-neglect (e.g. dehydration or starvation).

Treatment

Treatment can be:
- Pharmacological (antidepressants and mood stabilizers).
- Psychotherapeutic/social.
- Physical (ECT).

Both drug treatments and psychotherapy are effective in the treatment of depression. Prescribed at an adequate dose for a sufficiently long period (usually 6 weeks), with appropriate patient education and encouragement, an antidepressant will produce a remission in 60–70% of cases. When an antidepressant has brought remission of symptoms, it should be continued at full dose for at least 6 months to reduce the relapse rate.

A treatment may fail because a patient stopped taking the drug after unacceptable side effects or through a lack of response after 6 weeks at an adequate dose. Such failures should be addressed by the prescription of an alternative antidepressant from a different class. Antidepressants may fail for other reasons (see Chapter 15) such as non-compliance, which should be checked.

After three failures, depression is considered resistant and lithium augmentation (prescription of lithium in addition to an already prescribed tricyclic or SSRI) may be attempted.

Psychotic depression requires adjunctive use of an antipsychotic drug. When drug treatments have failed to induce remission, ECT may be used. ECT may be considered earlier for a depressed patient with psychomotor retardation.

Psychotherapeutic approaches (see Chapter 16) may be used as an alternative to medications or in combination with them. Options include:
- Cognitive therapy—challenges 'faulty' thoughts and assumptions.
- Behavioural therapy—attempts to modify behaviours that may lead to depression.
- Interpersonal therapy—concentrates on relationships, role disputes, losses, social deficits, and isolation.
- Psychoanalytic therapy—aims to change the personality structure by integrating repressed material from the past.

Pharmacotherapy is used in combination with simpler forms of psychotherapy in the outpatient-clinic setting, as a 'two-pronged' approach. Despite the limited time available in this setting, clinicians administering antidepressant treatment can encourage patients to explore their depression from a cognitive angle or to adopt behaviours that may protect against relapse.

BIPOLAR AFFECTIVE DISORDER

Aetiology
Biological and genetic factors
Most of the biological factors that have been suggested to have a role in depressive disorders may also be involved in bipolar affective disorder. The monoamine hypothesis is as applicable to elevated mood as it is to low mood, with manic episodes thought to be associated with increased central noradrenaline or serotonin.

Evidence from twin studies has again suggested a strong genetic component to the aetiology of bipolar affective disorder (more pronounced than in depression) and many patients have a positive family history.

Significant life events and severe stresses may provoke the onset of a first manic or hypomanic episode (e.g. there is an increased risk of manic episodes in the early postpartum period). However, there are no personality traits strongly associated with the development of bipolar affective disorder.

Epidemiology
Bipolar affective disorder is much less common than depression, the lifetime prevalence being around 1%, with no excess in females over males. Onset of manic episodes after the age of 50 years is unlikely and the mean age at first episode is considerably lower than in depression.

Investigations
As for depressive disorders, a battery of blood tests is normally performed on patients experiencing manic episodes to rule out an organic cause.

Course and prognosis
Around 85% of patients who go on to receive a diagnosis of bipolar affective disorder first experience a depressive episode; however, a small minority of bipolar patients never experience depressive episodes, having only periods of mania or hypomania between times of normality.

Manic episodes may last up to 3 months and tend to progress from expansiveness to eventual irritability. More than 90% of patients with bipolar affective disorder have more than one manic episode—some unfortunate individuals have as many as 20. In about 50% of cases, a second episode occurs within 2 years of the first. A minority develop 'rapid cycling', with four or more episodes a year—this is associated with a poor prognosis and a reported lifetime suicide risk of 10%.

Good prognostic factors in bipolar affective disorder are:
- Absence of comorbid psychiatric illness and alcohol abuse.
- Absence of depressive periods alternating with manic episodes.

Management setting
The initial management setting depends on the presentation and severity of illness. A manic episode may necessitate a period of hospitalization through:
- Reckless behaviour endangering the patient or others around them.
- Presence of psychotic symptoms.
- Disinhibited behaviour causing social taboos to be ignored.
- Indiscretions such as sexual impropriety and fiscal overspending.

Bipolar patients may also require hospital admission in depressive episodes for reasons outlined on page 154.

Treatment
Lithium is the drug of choice for prophylaxis and treatment in patients with bipolar affective disorder. Before commencing the drug, patients should be provided with information on its potential side effects and toxicity (see Chapter 16) and the need for periodic blood tests to assess the plasma level. As a mood-stabilizing agent, lithium successfully dampens down highs and lows in a majority of bipolar patients, providing adequate remission in about 55%. When effective, it should be continued for at least a year and may be maintained in the longer term as prophylaxis for any patient who has had more than one manic episode.

If lithium is introduced while a manic episode is in progress, it is usually necessary also to prescribe an antipsychotic for more immediate control of symptoms, as lithium itself usually takes days or weeks to produce therapeutic effects. In depressive episodes associated with bipolar affective disorder, antidepressants should be used with caution owing to a tendency to push mood beyond normal and provoke hypomanic or manic episodes.

When lithium fails through lack of efficacy or intolerance to side effects, the antiepileptic agent carbamazepine may be used as a second-line treatment. Sodium valproate is a further alternative.

Psychotherapy is performed much less commonly in bipolar affective disorder than in unipolar depression. Usually, patients referred for psychotherapy must be stabilized with lithium or an alternative agent, otherwise the therapy is unlikely to be productive.

CYCLOTHYMIA AND DYSTHYMIA

Aetiology
The extent to which the aetiologies of dysthymia and cyclothymia resemble those of depression and bipolar affective disorder is the subject of debate. There are biological similarities between dysthymia and depression; for example, REM latency is decreased in both conditions. Genetics link cyclothymia and bipolar affective disorder, as up to a third of patients with the former have a positive family history of the latter.

Epidemiology, course, and associations
Dysthymia is more common than cyclothymia, with a lifetime prevalence of 4% compared with 1%. Young people are at risk, with the majority of cyclothymics experiencing symptoms before their mid-twenties and dysthymia having an appreciable incidence in adolescence, although the low-grade but incessant nature of dysthymic symptoms is such that patients may take some years to reach the stage of requesting medical attention. Cyclothymia is slightly more common in females than males.

A third of patients with cyclothymia go on to suffer more severe affective disorders, most obviously bipolar affective disorder. Dysthymia may lead to depressive episodes and may coexist with anxiety disorders and borderline personality disorder.

Treatment
The two conditions may be treated pharmacologically with the same drugs used in depressive and bipolar affective disorder. Lithium and carbamazepine may be slightly more successful in cyclothymia than in bipolar illness, but antidepressants should be used with caution owing to their tendency to turn mild depressive symptoms into hypomania. SSRIs, MAOIs, and, sometimes, tricyclics can be used in dysthymia. Cognitive therapy can be used for both conditions.

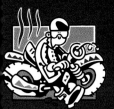

21. Anxiety and Somatoform Disorders

ANXIETY DISORDERS

These disorders are defined in Chapters 2, 3, and 4, and include:

- Generalized anxiety disorder.
- Panic disorder.
- Agoraphobia.
- Social phobia.
- Specific phobia.
- Obsessive–compulsive disorder.
- Post-traumatic stress disorder.

Aetiology

Genetic and biological factors

Genetic factors are thought to play some role in the development of most anxiety disorders.

Panic disorder and obsessive–compulsive disorder appear to be the most heritable anxiety disorders, with more than a third of those affected having a first-degree relative who has had the same diagnosis. The genetic contribution to generalized anxiety disorder is less clear-cut, but there is an association between this diagnosis and having relatives who abuse alcohol.

Biological factors have been the subject of considerable interest in anxiety disorders. Defects in neurotransmitter systems such as abnormal receptors may contribute to the development of specific disorders (e.g. generalized anxiety disorder—serotonin or GABA systems; panic disorder—serotonin, noradrenaline, or GABA). Obsessive-compulsive disorder is associated with a hypersensivity of some serotonin receptors, which is abolished by successful treatment with SSRIs.

Social and psychological factors

Anxiety disorders may be linked to the experience of stressors—in post-traumatic stress disorder a significant traumatic event is essential to the diagnosis, but stressors may precede the onset of symptoms in other anxiety disorders including panic disorder (recent marital separation) and agoraphobia.

Some psychiatrists take the view that anxiety disorders are predominantly psychological in origin.

Cognitive–behavioural theories suggest that symptoms and disorders are a consequence of inappropriate thought-processes and overestimation of dangers. Some examples of cognitive–behavioural theories for anxiety disorders are outlined below.

Panic attacks/panic disorder
A cognitive model of the panic attack suggests that an attack may be initiated when a susceptible individual misinterprets a normal body stimulus. For example: a patient may become aware of their heart beating; instead of dismissing this as normal, they may assume that it is under inordinate pressure and that something could be physically wrong; this fear may activate the sympathetic system, producing a real increase in the rate and strength of the heart beat; a vicious cycle may ensue, in which the perception of increasing cardiac effort convinces the sufferer that they are on the point of collapse or even myocardial infarction, leading to a crescendo of symptoms and then to a full-blown panic attack involving several of the panic symptoms listed in Chapter 2.

Specific phobias
Cognitive–behavioural theories of specific phobias hold that they are a consequence of childhood experiences in which exposure to something frightening occurs at the same time as exposure to a second object which would not normally provoke fear. The second object may itself become the focus of a phobia and can subsequently cause fear and avoidance. There appears to be an in-built predisposition for certain stimuli to be the focus of phobias rather than others—fear of spiders is far more common than fear of electricity sockets, yet contact with the latter poses a much greater risk to safety.

Post-traumatic stress disorder
Behavioural therapists may look at the link between an initial traumatic event and the subsequent flashbacks in terms of 'classical conditioning' (see Chapter 16) and the avoidance of situations which resemble that of the trauma as 'instrumental learning'.

Anxiety disorders may also be seen by psychoanalysts in terms of unresolved conflicts dating from childhood psychosexual development.

Epidemiology

Estimates of the prevalence of anxiety disorders (Fig. 21.1) are complicated by the fact that many people with such disorders are not diagnosed, either because they never present for treatment or because they present to medical specialists (e.g. to cardiologists when anxiety symptoms include palpitations and chest discomfort).

 Anxiety disorders are more common in women than in men except for social phobia and obsessive–compulsive disorder (where males and females are equally at risk) and post-traumatic stress disorder (where the sex ratio is not known).

Associations

Anxiety disorders often occur in tandem with other psychiatric disorders (Fig. 21.2); for example, 50% of patients with generalized anxiety disorder experience at least one other psychiatric disorder in their lifetime.

Although anxiety disorders—especially generalized anxiety disorder and panic disorder—feature physical symptoms that may mimic medical problems such as thyrotoxicosis and phaeochromocytoma, there are also some physical diseases that may be comorbid with, or secondary to, anxiety disorders:

- Panic disorder is associated with hypertension, and panic disorder patients are prone to excess mortality through cardiovascular causes. It was previously thought that panic disorder was associated with prolapse of the mitral valve, but subsequent research has shown that this is not the case.
- Obsessive–compulsive disorder patients who exhibit compulsive hand washing may suffer dermatological problems.

Investigations

The anxiety disorders described here can only be diagnosed when the symptoms are not due to the direct effect of a substance or general medical

Fig. 21.1 Lifetime prevalence, sex, and age distribution of anxiety disorders.

Lifetime prevalence, sex, and age distribution of anxiety disorders			
Disorder	**Lifetime prevalence**	**Sex ratio**	**Most common age at onset**
generalized anxiety disorder	7%	f>m	20s/30s
panic disorder	5%	f>m (3:1)	20s/30s
obsessive–compulsive disorder	2%	f=m	under 25 years
post-traumatic stress disorder	2%*	unknown	(any age)
social phobia	15%**	f=m	teenage years
specific phobia		f>m	10–15 years
agoraphobia		f>m (3:1)	20s/30s

* A further 10% of the population may experience some symptoms suggestive of post traumatic stress disorder but fail to meet the criteria for the diagnosis
**Combined lifetime prevalence for social phobia, specific phobia, and agoraphobia. Specific phobia is the most common among these disorders

condition. This stipulation is particularly relevant when considering diagnoses of generalized anxiety disorder and panic disorder.

It is of course impractical to test for each of the large number of drugs and organic conditions capable of producing anxiety symptoms (see Fig. 2.5). It is however important to exclude any disease or substance that may be implicated through any clues in the history (e.g. past medical history and drug history) and physical examination. For example, a patient with exophthalmos should have thyroid function tests in case thyrotoxicosis is provoking apparent anxiety symptoms. The possibility of withdrawal syndromes (e.g. alcohol, benzodiazepines, narcotics) causing anxiety symptoms should also be considered.

Course and prognosis

The prognoses of anxiety disorders vary greatly between individuals.

Examples of psychiatric conditions associated with anxiety disorders	
Disorder	**Psychiatric condition**
generalized anxiety disorder	depression other anxiety disorders alcohol/substance misuse
panic disorder	agoraphobia and other anxiety disorders depression (>50% lifetime risk) alcohol/substance misuse suicide
obsessive–compulsive disorder	depression suicide Gilles de la Torrette's syndrome*
post-traumatic stress disorder	depression other anxiety disorders alcohol/substance misuse borderline personality disorder
social** and specific phobias	alcohol misuse

* The majority of patients with this tic disorder fulfil the criteria for obsessive–compulsive disorder
**Social phobia may be secondary to depression through low self-esteem

Fig. 21.2 Examples of psychiatric conditions associated with anxiety disorders.

Depending on treatment, up to one-half of panic disorder patients may be symptom-free after 3 years, but one-third of the remainder have chronic symptoms that are sufficiently distressing to significantly reduce quality of life. Panic attacks are central to the development of agoraphobia, and progression to other psychiatric disorders is common.

Generalized anxiety is more likely to be chronic, especially if the original episode lasts for more than 6 months. Other poor prognostic features are severe symptoms, agitation, derealization, and episodes of fainting.

Obsessive–compulsive disorder may also be long lasting in up to a third of patients, who remain incapacitated by their symptoms in spite of treatment. This outcome is associated with early onset, need for hospitalization, and comorbid depression.

Similarly, approximately one-third of patients with post-traumatic stress disorder are left with moderate to severe symptoms in the long term, but a greater proportion achieve full recovery—this is most likely when the symptoms arrive within 6 months of the trauma and no other psychiatric illnesses are present.

The long-term prognosis of phobias is less well known, but it is thought that simple phobias that persist from childhood are less likely to remit than those that begin in response to distress in adulthood.

In post-traumatic stress disorder, the time lag between the original traumatic event and the onset of symptoms is usually a matter of weeks or months but can be many years.

Management setting

Most anxiety disorders can be treated in outpatient departments or day hospitals. However, admission to an inpatient unit is sometimes required—for example, in:

- Severe obsessive–compulsive disorder.
- Panic disorder with severe agoraphobia.

Treatment

Most anxiety disorders can be treated by drugs or by psychotherapy, or by a combination of the two (Fig. 21.3).

The finding that antidepressants can produce a remission of panic attacks in most patients with panic disorder but have little effect on generalized anxiety disorder led to the two conditions being recognized as distinct disorders. Antidepressants are generally prescribed at lower doses for panic disorder than for depression. SSRIs and clomipramine have a strong record of efficacy in obsessive–compulsive disorder.

Benzodiazepines are useful in treatment of generalized anxiety disorder and, at higher doses, panic disorder. Although they will provide faster relief than antidepressants in panic disorder, their value in both conditions is limited by the propensity to tolerance, addiction, and withdrawal symptoms on discontinuation. Alternatives in generalized anxiety disorder include short-term antipsychotics (best reserved for severe anxiety) and new drugs such as buspirone.

Beta blockers (e.g. propanolol) may be useful in combating the autonomic symptoms of anxiety in both generalized anxiety disorder and panic disorder, such as racing pulse and sweating.

Fig. 21.3 Treatment of anxiety disorders.

Treatment of anxiety disorders		
Disorder	**Drug treatments**	**Non-drug treatment**
generalized anxiety disorder	benzodiazepines antipsychotics (for severe anxiety) buspirone beta blockers	cognitive–behavioural therapy supportive therapy psychodynamic therapy
panic disorder/agoraphobia	antidepressants • tricyclics • SSRIs • MAOIs benzodiazepines (alprazolam) beta blockers	cognitive–behavioural therapy (including exposure) relaxation training
social phobia	antidepressants • SSRIs • MAOIs benzodiazepines beta blockers	cognitive–behavioural therapy
specific phobia	—	cognitive–behavioural therapy (including exposure) psychodynamic (insight-orientated) therapy
obsessive–compulsive disorder	antidepressants • SSRIs and clomipramine • some MAOIs	cognitive–behavioural therapy supportive and family therapy
post-traumatic stress disorder	antidepressants • tricyclics • SSRIS • MAOIS	psychodynamic therapy cognitive–behavioural therapy (including exposure)

MAOIs=monoamine oxidase inhibitors
SSRIs=selective serotonin reuptake inhibitors

Cognitive–behavioural therapy is effective for many anxiety disorders (see Fig. 21.3). For specific phobias and post-traumatic stress disorder, a form known as exposure therapy, which involves gradual desensitization to a feared object or situation, is used (see Chapter 16).

In panic disorder, cognitive–behavioural therapy may involve helping the sufferer to understand that a panic attack may start from a misinterpretation of a normal stimulus, leading to a 'vicious cycle' of spiralling fear and sympathetic activation. When the patient understands this model, the therapist may encourage the patient to break the cycle by promoting rejection of the assumption that the original stimulus (e.g. palpitations) is indicative of impending physical dysfunction (e.g.heart attack).

Other therapies commonly used in anxiety disorders are supportive, psychodynamic, and family therapies (see Chapter 16).

SOMATOFORM DISORDERS

These disorders are defined in Chapter 9 and include:
- Somatization disorder.
- Somatoform pain disorder.
- Hypochondriasis.
- Conversion disorders.

Aetiology

The aetiology of somatoform disorders is poorly understood, although episodes often follow the appearance of a stressor. In the case of somatoform pain disorder, the stressor typically involves pain (e.g. unexpected physical trauma).

Somatization disorder may have some genetic component in that up to one-fifth of sufferers' female first-degree relatives also have the condition. Theories of a biological aetiology include the suggestion that physical symptoms result from a failure to regulate cytokines (e.g. interleukins). Psychological models consider the symptoms to be produced as a surrogate form of communication.

Patients with hypochondriasis may simply have a lower threshold for identifying illness or may subconsciously covet the gains to be had from adopting the sick role.

Epidemiology

Somatization disorder has a lifetime prevalence of less than 0.5%.

There are no data on the lifetime prevalence of hypochondriasis or somatoform pain disorder, but both disorders are common among patients who present recurrently in primary care.

Conversion disorders are considerably more rare. Using the DSM-IV definition, which restricts conversion disorders to the experience of neurological symptoms of no organic basis following stress, the prevalence is only one-tenth that of somatization disorder. Dissociative states such as dissociative amnesia, fugue, and stupor are also rare.

Somatization disorder usually starts before the age of 30—in some classifications this is essential. The onset of hypochondriasis, by contrast, may be at any age, although the peak incidence is between 20 and 30. The age of onset of somatoform pain disorder is also very variable, but is most likely to occur between 30 and 40. While somatization disorder is linked with low socioeconomic status, hypochondriasis is equally common in all socioeconomic groups.

Associations

All somatoform disorders are associated with the presence of personality disorders (e.g. avoidant, obsessive–compulsive) or dysfunctional personality traits.

Somatization disorder and hypochondriasis frequently occur in association with generalized anxiety disorder, phobias, and depressive disorders. Hypochondriasis is also associated with schizophrenia.

Females outnumber males by up to 20:1 in somatization disorder, but there is no sex difference in the prevalence of hypochondriasis.

Course and prognosis

Both somatization disorder and hypochondriasis tend to have a chronic episodic course: episodes—which are often provoked by stressors—may go on for many months before a period of remission is reached. Patients with hypochondriasis are more likely to achieve a full remission; good prognostic features include the absence of a personality disorder and a diagnosed medical problem, and the presence of a psychiatric disorder that responds to treatment (e.g. depression).

Conversion disorders usually resolve quickly and spontaneously, and symptoms recur in only a quarter of cases.

Treatment

Patients who complain of many symptoms or illnesses may seek to present to a variety of doctors in different specialties. It is therefore desirable for one doctor, often the general practitioner, to take charge of the patient's case so that a coordinated judgement can be made as new features appear. Mindful that patients with diagnosed somatoform disorders can still go on to experience medical problems, the responsible clinician must evaluate the presentation of new symptoms or claims of further illnesses carefully, with physical examination and simple tests as indicated, but he or she must also be aware that specialist referral for every symptom may be counterproductive.

Drug treatment is indicated for comorbid psychiatric illness such as anxiety and depression. Supportive psychotherapy may prove valuable and should aim to help the patient to deal with symptoms (rather than trying to convince them that the symptoms are 'all in the mind').

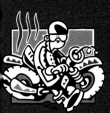

22. Eating, Sleep, and Sexual Disorders, and Disorders of the Puerperium

EATING DISORDERS

This chapter will discuss anorexia nervosa and bulimia nervosa, and atypical forms of these disorders. Definitions were presented in Chapter 10.

Aetiology

There are many theories about the aetiology of eating disorders. Biological theories involve noradrenaline or endorphins (anorexia and bulimia) and serotonin [bulimia—in line with the efficacy of the selective serotonin reuptake inhibitor (SSRI) fluoxetine in treating this disorder].

Anorexia nervosa

Anorexia nervosa may represent a desire to escape the pressures of growing up in individuals who are psychosexually immature, or a desire to compensate for low self-esteem by exerting a rigid control over the body. It appears to be more common in children of close families of higher socioeconomic status, and depression is more common in relatives of those affected. The importance of genetics is debatable, despite evidence that siblings of anorexia nervosa patients are at much increased risk, as this may reflect family behaviour (e.g. emphasis within the family group on diet and exercise) rather than genetics. Peer-group pressure to diet and enmeshed family interactions have also been implicated.

Bulimia nervosa

In contrast to the extreme control over the body in anorexia nervosa, bulimia is associated with a loss of control. Binge eating may provide transient relief in response to low mood, anxiety, or distressing events, but after the induction of vomiting the relief soon gives way to guilt, or further depressive symptoms and anxiety.

As with anorexia, bulimia nervosa is associated with depression in family members, but families are typically less close-knit and there is less of an association with socioeconomic status. Individuals with bulimia are often eloquent and sociable people who have achieved success in their education but have a tendency to impulsive behaviour. They may find it difficult to maintain relationships and some have borderline personality traits. Like patients with anorexia nervosa, they may have low self-esteem and comorbid depression, and are additionally prone to abuse of alcohol and drug addiction.

A notable minority of patients with anorexia nervosa and bulimia nervosa were actually overweight (body mass index >25 kg/m^2) before development of their symptoms. Such individuals may have been overly exposed to society's encouragement to achieve a slim figure and sought to prolong initial compliments gained on achieving appropriate weight loss.

There is considerable overlap between symptoms of anorexia nervosa and bulimia nervosa, especially when anorexic patients who lose weight by purging and vomiting rather than by restricting intake are considered. The main diagnostic difference is that patients with anorexia nervosa must be grossly underweight (see Chapter 10). Remember also that a proportion of patients who originally have anorexia nervosa go on to fulfil the criteria for bulimia nervosa.

Epidemiology

Anorexia nervosa is predominantly a disease of young caucasian women (the female to male ratio is more

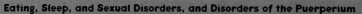

than 10:1). Its onset is usually in the teenage years, peaking at 17 years, and almost always between the ages of 10 and 35 years. Estimates of prevalence in adolescent females are 0.2–1.0%. It is more common among high socioeconomic groups.

Bulimia nervosa is more common, with a prevalence in young females of 1.5–2.5%. The peak age of onset is later than in anorexia; onset is often after adolescence is completed. Males are rarely affected.

Complications

Physiological changes associated with excessive weight loss and with purging and vomiting are listed in Chapter 10. Both anorexia nervosa and bulimia nervosa may provoke secondary depression, which, if severe, can carry a suicide risk.

Investigations

A physical examination is important in assessing patients with eating disorders, to quantify physical changes associated with reduced nutritional intake (e.g. dehydration, emaciation, alteration of hair distribution) or purging (dental caries, enlargement of parotid glands).

Laboratory investigations are indicated in assessment of such patients, firstly, to exclude organic causes of weight loss (e.g. blood glucose for diabetes mellitus, thyroid function tests for hyperthyroidism), and secondly, to examine the extent of physiological changes associated with starvation or vomiting. Investigations for the latter comprise:

- Electrolytes—it is especially important to measure these in cases of repeated vomiting because this may be associated with loss of potassium and metabolic alkalosis. Abuse of diuretics may also cause hypokalaemia.
- Urea and creatinine (for renal function) and ECG— these are valuable in pronounced hypokalaemia, which can provoke renal damage or cardiac arrhythmias.
- Full blood count (to exclude leucopaenia).
- Mineral levels (to assess need for vitamin replacement).

Course and prognosis

Of the two main eating disorders, anorexia nervosa has the poorer prognosis. The outcome is highly variable:

- Approximately 20% recover fully—some without needing treatment.

- Approximately 20% experience chronic severe illness, and, in long-term follow-up, 10–15% die prematurely by suicide or complications of starvation and electrolyte disturbance.
- The rest may recover partially but may fluctuate and relapse and, in spite of returning to acceptable weight, show ongoing psychological problems.

Note that around 40% of anorexic patients develop bulimic symptoms at some point in their illness.

Outcome is generally better in bulimia nervosa, with the majority who have antidepressants or psychotherapy having a full or partial response. The disease can run a chronic relapsing course and a minority of patients require periods of hospitalization for medical reasons (especially electrolyte imbalance through repeated vomiting).

Treatment
Anorexia nervosa

Patients with anorexia nervosa may be treated as outpatients or inpatients. Inpatient treatment may be needed in the presence of one or more of the following:

- Extensive or rapid weight loss.
- Poor physical health, either predating anorexia nervosa or as a direct result of starvation or purging.
- Severe depressive features with or without suicidality.
- Need for a supportive structure not adequately provided in an outpatient setting.

Ideally, hospitalization should be planned in advance, with the patient and therapist agreeing on a programme of gradual weight gain—but to even reach this stage of agreement, some anorexic patients may require considerable education and encouragement.

Sometimes, hospital admission is indicated as an emergency. A patient with severe weight loss, accompanied perhaps by dehydration and potentially electrolyte disturbance, may be at a considerable health risk – even at risk of death.

The mainstay of treatment is behavioural therapy backed up by vigilant and supportive nursing. The aim is to introduce a progressively higher calorific intake, with close monitoring of weight each day, in pursuit of an approximate target weight (body mass index of 18 or more, depending on build and original weight). Food is initially divided into several small meals per day (so as not to appear too daunting) and may be supplemented by high-calorie drinks. Nursing staff are trained to praise the patient when appropriate but also to ensure that recourse to strategies that may counteract weight gain (exercise, vomiting, laxative use) is prevented or challenged.

Family therapy (see Chapter 24), cognitive therapy (which may challenge dysfunctional beliefs about ideal weight), and dynamic therapy may be used to support inpatient or outpatient treatment and can be continued after a target weight is reached. Drug treatment has provided little benefit in anorexia nervosa, other than for symptomatic relief of anxiety symptoms.

Bulimia nervosa

Patients with bulimia nervosa tend to accept treatment more readily than those with anorexia nervosa and most can be managed in outpatients unless they have comorbid depression of sufficient severity to require hospitalization or are actively suicidal.

Drug therapy is more effective in bulimia than in anorexia, with the SSRI fluoxetine now licensed for treatment at a 60 mg daily dose (higher than that used in depression). Its efficacy in reducing bingeing and purging is not dependent on the presence of depression, anxiety, or other comorbid psychiatric disorders. Tricyclics and monoamine oxidase inhibitors (MAOIs) have also been used with success in bulimia, and, when bulimia coexists with depression, use of antidepressants can potentially ameliorate both disorders.

Cognitive–behavioural therapy, focusing on thoughts and behaviour before and during a session of overeating, is similarly effective in reducing bingeing and vomiting. The other psychotherapies used for anorexia nervosa (dynamic and family therapy) may also have a place in treatment of bulimia nervosa.

SLEEP DISORDERS

Insomnia

Insomnia (difficulty in getting to sleep or staying asleep, or non-refreshing sleep) may be experienced by up to one-third of the general population.

Aetiology

The causes of insomnia are listed in Fig. 10.1.

Insomnia is:

- 'Primary' in 15% of cases.
- Secondary to other psychiatric disorders (e.g. depression , anxiety disorders) in 30–40%.
- Secondary to alcohol, medications, or other psychoactive substances (e.g. caffeine) in 10–15%.
- Secondary to medical conditions (e.g. chronic pain) in 10%.
- Secondary to specific sleep syndromes (e.g. sleep apnoea, restless-legs syndromes, disorders of the sleep–wake schedule) in 15%.

Depression may be associated with 'early morning wakening'—a characteristic form of insomnia in which the patient wakes very early in the morning and is subsequently unable to resume sleep. However, about one-fifth of depressed patients who report sleep problems complain of hypersomnia.

Investigations and treatment

When treating a patient complaining of insomnia, it is essential to exclude any possible psychiatric, medical, or substance-related cause before proceeding to more sleep-specific investigations. It is notoriously difficult to take a reliable sleep history from insomniacs, as they may greatly misjudge the number and length of awakenings and the time spent asleep. However, sleep architecture—the sleep pattern, including rapid eye movement (REM) sleep, stages I–IV of non-REM sleep, and awakenings—can be investigated using 16-lead EEG recording, with the patient spending the night in the investigation suite or at home.

Primary or non-organic insomnia is difficult to treat satisfactorily. Initial measures include aiming to improve sleep hygiene, i.e.:

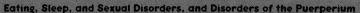

- Encouraging regular time for sleep.
- Ensuring the bedroom is quiet and comfortable.
- Using the bedroom only for sleep (and sexual activity), not for work or hobbies.
- Using a regular sleep cue.

A healthy diet (avoiding excess caffeine, especially later in the day) and regular exercise may also help.

As normal sleep should be initiated within 10 minutes, patients who have not fallen asleep within about 15 minutes are encouraged to get up and pursue a different activity (deconditioning) and try sleeping later. Other forms of psychotherapy are generally ineffective.

When insomnia occurs with depression, a sedative tricyclic antidepressant may provide immediate improvement in sleep. It is said that SSRIs improve sleep more gradually, in parallel with their action in relieving low mood.

Hypnotic drugs—such as benzodiazepines (temazepam, nitrazepam), chloral hydrate, zopiclone, and zolpidem—should be prescribed with caution. Their varying associations with tolerance and difficult withdrawal (especially the benzodiazepines)—see Chapter 15—means that they should be prescribed on a time-limited basis (e.g. 2–4 weeks), ideally for use on alternate or occasional nights rather than every night.

Hypersomnia and narcolepsy

Hypersomnia is much less common than insomnia. Again, it may be primary or it may be secondary to medical or psychiatric conditions, substance-related causes, or specific sleep syndromes— in particular, narcolepsy.

Aetiology

Narcolepsy is a condition of excess daytime somnolence with sleep attacks, caused by an abnormality of mechanisms that inhibit REM sleep. It may be associated with cataplexy (sudden loss of muscle tone, sometimes with a short-lived paralysis). Hypnogogic and hypnopompic hallucinations— apparently-abnormal perceptions that occur in normal individuals as they move from sleep to wakefulness— may be very pronounced in narcolepsy.

Epidemiology

Narcolepsy usually begins in the teenage years or twenties, and tends to run a chronic course. It affects 0.1% of adults, males more than females. There is a definite genetic component as most narcoleptics carry the HLA-DR2 antigen and one-third have a family history with apparent autosomal dominant inheritance in such lines. The diagnosis can be confirmed by EEG recording (looking for immediate onset of REM) or by timing sleep latency.

Treatment

Narcoleptics can be assisted by adopting a lifestyle that allows for planned daytime 'power naps'. Sleep attacks may be brought on by stress—thus, stressors should be identified and avoided, and activities such as driving may be contraindicated. Amphetamines may offer some benefit and tricyclic antidepressants have been used to treat the cataplexy component.

Sleep apnoea syndromes

Aetiology

In sleep apnoea syndromes, entry of air is episodically blocked at the nose or mouth, resulting in 'apnoeic periods' and brief arousal. There may be many such arousals each night, and, although they are not recalled, the refreshing quality of sleep is much reduced. Thus, patients may compensate through daytime somnolence or even sleep attacks. Sleep partners may report episodic periods of loud snoring, and may even observe the patient apparently stop breathing.

Epidemiology

Sleep apnoea affects males more than females and is more prevalent in those over 35. The overall prevalence is not known, but onset is often associated with weight gain, because deposition of facial fat increases the likelihood of anatomical obstruction.

Investigations

The diagnosis of sleep apnoea can be confirmed by admission for a night to a specialist bed where EEG and oxygen-saturation recordings are made. Weight loss may be recommended as an initial treatment, but more direct relief can be gained from a CPAP (continuous positive airways pressure) mask, which can be worn at night to ensure the airway is kept open. Nasal surgery is also an option. As in narcolepsy, patients should be advised against driving whilst affected by the condition, given the disastrous consequences of suffering a sleep attack at the wheel.

DISORDERS OF SEXUALITY

Sexual dysfunction

The symptoms of sexual dysfunctions in males and females are discussed in Chapter 10. The dysfunctions are summarized in Fig. 22.1.

Aetiology

Sexual dysfunction may be caused by:

- Organic factors, such as a general medical condition (see Fig. 10.2) or drug side effects (see Fig. 10.3).
- Psychological factors.
- A combination of both.

Psychological factors that may underlie sexual dysfunction include:

- Lack of knowledge about sexual techniques.
- Anxiety about sexual performance (especially if there have been previous failures or when a relationship is under strain).
- Previous distressing experience such as rape or abuse.
- Diminishing interest in, or affection for, sexual partner.
- Comorbid psychiatric illness (e.g. depression causing loss of sexual interest as a biological symptom).

For instance, between 25–50% of men with erectile dysfunction have an organic cause such as diabetes, hypothroidism, or treatment with drugs such as thiazide diuretics (e.g. bendrofluazide) or sedating antidepressants (e.g. amitriptyline). The aetiology may be purely psychological for reasons such as marital strain, or the dysfunction may be related to depression. Erectile dysfunction may be due to a combination of any of these factors—for example, a patient with angina may develop 'performance anxiety' or lose interest in intercourse altogether, through fear that sexual activity will provoke an attack necessitating premature abandonment.

Dyspareunia is usually caused by organic factors (e.g. endometriosis), but may develop from vaginisimus, which is most often a psychological reaction to fears about intercourse. Conversely, vaginisimus may follow development of dyspareunia.

Epidemiology

Reliable estimations of the prevalence of sexual dysfunctions are scarce, with great variations in results owing to the use of differing criteria and methods of assessment. However, it is known that females outnumber males in dysfunctions of sexual desire and that, relatively speaking, hypoactive sexual desire is much more common than sexual aversion disorder.

Erectile dysfunction in the male (impotence) may be lifelong or acquired. The lifetime prevalence is around 15%. Risk of problems with sexual arousal increase with age but may not merit diagnosis in the elderly if sexual activity has ceased. Disorders of sexual arousal in the female are probably common but underdiagnosed.

Classification of sexual dysfunction in females and males		
Dysfunction category	Female	Male
sexual desire disorders	hypoactive sexual desire sexual aversion	hypoactive sexual desire sexual aversion
sexual arousal disorders	female sexual arousal disorder	erectile dysfunction
orgasm disorders	anorgasmia (female orgasmic disorder)	male orgasmic disorder premature ejaculation
sexual pain disorders	dyspareunia vaginisimus	dyspareunia

Fig. 22.1 Classification of sexual dysfunction in females and males.

Female orgasmic disorder is the most common sexual dysfunction in women presenting to psychosexual clinics. A small proportion of females may never achieve orgasm, but the acquired disorder may have a lifetime prevalence of over 25%. The prevalence of orgasm disorder in the male is much lower, around 5%.

Premature ejaculation is second only to erectile dysfunction as the main complaint of men presenting with sexual disorders. In contrast to erectile dysfunction, it is more common in younger men, being particularly common in those having their first sexual relationships.

Vaginisimus is associated with high socioeconomic status and, by definition, is seen only in females. Dyspareunia can occur in either sex but is much more common in women. The overall prevalences of these conditions are not known.

Investigations

Many large cities provide a specific clinic where partners with marital and sexual difficulties can be jointly assessed. A full medical and psychiatric history is required and clinicians must be alert to identifying both organic and psychological factors that may underlie a sexual dysfunction.

A routine screen to rule out common organic disorders includes a full blood count, urea and electrolytes, glucose, liver, and thyroid function tests, and other hormonal assays. In assessing erectile dysfunction, penile blood flow (internal pudendal artery) can be measured using a Doppler flow meter.

Investigation of dyspareunia in the female requires specialist gynaecological examination (e.g. for retroversion of the uterus).

Course and prognosis

Vaginisimus has the best outcome, especially when psychotherapy is undertaken, whereas disorders of sexual desire have the least encouraging prognosis and tend to be chronic. If an organic factor is largely responsible for a sexual dysfunction, the prognosis depends on the degree to which the specific organic disorder is amenable to treatment.

Treatment

Disorders of sexual dysfunction may be treated by :
- Psychotherapy.
- Specific exercises.
- Drug therapy.
- Surgical therapy.

Psychotherapy can be applied to any sexual dysfunction disorder when the predominant cause is thought not to be organic. Therapy normally involves both partners and may involve both a male and a female therapist. Behavioural therapies in which changes in the pattern of sexual behaviour are discussed and subsequently attempted at home are most commonly used.

Examples of exercises used to ameliorate symptoms of sexual dysfunction are:
- The squeeze technique in premature ejaculation, whereby the female squeezes the penis prior to ejaculation, thus delaying its impending onset.
- Self-induced progressive dilatation of the vagina for vaginisimus.

Drug therapy is most useful to treat:
- General medical conditions responsible for sexual dysfunction.
- Underlying or comorbid mental illness, such as anxiety disorders and depression, which may contribute to sexual dysfunction—a tricyclic antidepressant prescribed to a depressed man with premature ejaculation may not only treat mood but also provide more direct benefit through its side effect of causing delay of orgasm.

> **Erectile and orgasmic dysfunctions are more likely to be psychological in origin if they occur with one specific partner but are absent either on intercourse with another partner or on masturbation. A male with erectile dysfunction who is nevertheless capable of morning or other spontaneous erections is also unlikely to have an organic cause.**

Evidence for drugs claimed to treat sexual dysfunctions specifically is generally disappointing, but intercavernosal injection of alprostadil (prostaglandin E1) has been licensed in the UK for treatment of erectile dysfunction. A side effect of this treatment is priapism— prolongation of erection for more than 4 hours, requiring urgent treatment by aspiration or injection of sympathomimetics. Papaverine (a smooth muscle relaxant) with or without phentolamine is also used for erectile dysfunction but is not licensed in the UK.

Another drug yet to be licensed in this country is Viagra® (sildenafil), a phosphodiesterase 5 inhibator administered orally. Evidence from clinical trails suggest that sildenafil may be a convenient and effective therapy for men with erectile dysfunction.

Surgical therapy is appropriate for sexual dysfunctions, including those due to a certain organic cause. Examples are vascular shunts to optimize penile blood flow (erectile dysfunction), fitting of penile prostheses, and remodelling of the vagina or hymen (poor sensation or dyspareunia). Unfortunately, evidence of success is limited. Other therapies for erectile dysfunction include vacuum erection devices and urethral inserts.

Disorders of sexual preference (paraphilias)

In paraphilias (Fig. 22.2), the object of sexual arousal or the behaviour used to achieve sexual arousal is abnormal.

Aetiology

Most paraphilias are thought to be a consequence of inhibition of the development of heterosexual desires. In individuals who are shy or fearful of heterosexual relationships, fetishism may be caused by chance associations of inanimate objects with sexual arousal which persist to override heterosexual impulses.

Behaviour involving the fulfilment of paraphilic urges may be provoked by psychiatric illness (e.g. depression, manic episodes in bipolar affective disorder, schizophrenia, and alcoholism). In older men, the behaviour may be associated with onset of dementia or other organic disease.

Epidemiology

Disorders of sexual preference are mainly confined to males (with the exception of sexual masochism) and usually begin in late adolescence or early adulthood. As paedophila and exhibitionism may involve the abuse of children, these conditions are often seen in a forensic setting, and account for the majority of sexual offenders referred for a psychiatric opinion. Exhibitionism is associated with antisocial (dissocial) personality disorder and with dementia. The prevalence of paraphilias in the general population is not known.

Fig. 22.2 Classification of paraphilias.

Classification of paraphilias	
Paraphilia	**Object/behaviour**
exhibitionism	public exposure of genitals
fetishism	inanimate objects (usually associated with the body)
frotteurism	rubbing against others in crowded spaces
paedophilia	genital fondling or further sexual acts with prepubescent children (may be limited to fantasy only)
sexual masochism	humiliation, beating, or other suffering by a sexual partner
sexual sadism	beating or causing humiliation or suffering to a sexual partner
fetishistic transvestism	cross-dressing
voyeurism	surreptitious observation of another who is naked or having intercourse

Investigations, treatment, and prognosis

When patients with sexual-preference disorders are referred to psychiatrists, it is essential for any other psychiatric and organic conditions to be identified and treated appropriately.

Drug treatment is limited. Antiandrogens (e.g. cyproterone acetate) have been used with some success to dampen sexual drive. Psychotherapy, including cognitive–behavioural techniques, has been attempted to encourage heterosexual urges and expression at the expense of the paraphilia and to promote insight into the development of the disorder. Generally, however, paraphilias persist for long periods, especially when they start at an early age and do not provoke guilt or a desire for change.

DISORDERS OF THE PUERPERIUM

The three main syndromes encountered in the puerperium are defined in Chapter 10 and comprise:
- 'Baby blues'.
- Postnatal depression (and other non-psychotic illnesses such as generalized anxiety disorder and phobias).
- Puerperal psychosis.

Aetiology and risk factors

The mild disturbance of mood experienced in baby blues may be a biological or psychosocial consequence of childbirth. Dramatic alterations in hormone levels provide a biological explanation. The stress of going through the delivery, along with feelings of new responsibilities associated with a baby's arrival, are obvious psychological factors.

Postnatal depression and puerperal psychosis may represent more marked reactions to the same biological or psychological factors. Hormonal changes may be exacerbated by oversensitivity of receptors to change, and, in individuals with a propensity to mood disorder, psychological stressors may strain coping mechanisms to excess.

Risk factors for puerperal psychosis are:
- History of bipolar affective disorder.
- Previous puerperal psychosis.
- Primiparous mother.

- Delivery associated with obstetric complications, caesarean section, or perinatal death.
- Family history of depression or affective disorders.
- Marriage problems during pregnancy.

Occasionally, puerperal psychosis has an organic aetiology, through cortical effects of eclampsia, low blood volume, or perinatal infection, or side effects of medications administered around the time of delivery.

Epidemiology

As expected, the prevalence of the three conditions is inversely related to their severity. For example:
- More than one in three deliveries are followed by a period of self-limiting 'baby blues'.
- Postnatal depression occurs after one in eight deliveries.
- Puerperal psychosis is rare, occurring after fewer than 1 per 500 pregnancies.

 The incidence of psychiatric illness (excluding non-pathological blues) is increased by five to seven times in puerperal women compared with non-puerperal controls. The risk of psychiatric admission in the 30 days after delivery of a first child is 35 times that prior to pregnancy.

Course and prognosis

Baby blues are self-limiting, symptoms usually resolving within 10 days. Sometimes, apparent baby blues herald the onset of more severe postnatal depression.

In postnatal depression, the depressive features are usually established within 2–4 weeks of the birth. Like any depressive episode, it can last several months if untreated, but appropriate treatment should provide remission in 4–6 weeks.

Onset of symptoms of puerperal psychosis may be within days or may be delayed for up to 6 weeks, and initially features may resemble postnatal depression. Recovery from an acute episode of puerperal psychosis is normally complete within 3 months, but a risk of recurrence of up to 20% is carried into future pregnancies, and there is a risk of recurrence of the underlying disorder (usually depressive or bipolar) within a year after the birth.

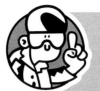

Tricyclics, SSRIs, MAOIs, and antipsychotics are not contraindicated in breastfeeding women, but manufacturers advise caution. Note that breastfeeding mothers should not be given benzodiazepines on a regular basis as the quantities passed to the baby are sufficient to cause lethargy and weight loss.

Investigations and treatment

Baby blues requires no treatment beyond normal postpartum support. However, women experiencing such symptoms should be observed carefully in case the symptoms persist and develop into a depressive episode.

Management of the more severe disorders involves thorough communication with both parents and with all professionals involved in postnatal care. Postnatal depression should be treated with medication and counselling in a similar fashion to a non-puerperal depressive episode. Bottle-feeding may be preferable to breastfeeding in these circumstances—to allow the duty of feeding to be shared and to avoid the possibility of antidepressants reaching the neonate through the breast milk.

Puerperal psychosis requires emergency treatment. The possibility of symptoms being provoked by eclampsia or sepsis should be ruled out—in liaison with the gynaecologists if necessary. Antidepressants or antipsychotics may be used (with the caveats above). Lithium may be required for a predominantly manic psychosis, if breastfeeding is avoided. The condition is associated with suicide and infanticide and the risk is usually sufficient to necessitate the mother's admission to a psychiatric unit—in some centres mother-and-baby places are available. Separation of mother and baby may be necessary, especially when content of delusions or hallucinations point to the possibility of harming the child, but closely supervised contact is generally allowed in the interest of bonding.

Psychotherapy may be provided both for puerperal psychosis patients who have recovered from their initial psychotic episode and for postnatal depressives who have failed to respond to either antidepressants or counselling. Cognitive–behavioural therapy is of proven value in the latter group.

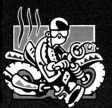

23. Personality Disorders

PERSONALITY DISORDERS AND TRAITS

Personality disorders are ingrained patterns of behaviour, emotion, or internal experience which deviate from the social and cultural norm and cause distress or impairment of functioning. Deviant personality characteristics that exist without causing such problems are known as personality traits.

Features of personality disorders are as follows:
- Their roots are in adolescence or childhood.
- They remain constant over years (but not necessarily over a lifetime) in spite of mood fluctuations.
- They give rise to a behaviour pattern recognizable by others.

There are some differences in the personality disorder categories between ICD-10 and DSM-IV (Fig. 23.1). For full descriptions, see Chapter 8.

Other known personality disorders such as passive–aggressive personality disorder and depressive personality disorder appear in a 'not otherwise specified' category in DSM-IV but are not listed in ICD-10.

Aetiology
Psychological factors are thought to play an important role in personality traits and disorders. For example, childhood sexual abuse may lead to the development of borderline personality disorder. Defence mechanisms (e.g. splitting, dissociation, projection) may assist the patient to live without guilt, shame, fear, or anxiety and produce behaviour that is ego-syntonic—viewed as satisfactory and helpful to the individual irrespective of distress it may cause to others.

There is evidence of some genetic basis to personality disorders through both twin studies and observations of family associations between those with personality disorders and those with certain mental illnesses. For example:
- Schizotypal and possibly paranoid personality disorders are more prevalent in relatives of schizophrenics.

- Borderline personality disorder is associated with a family history of depression.

Evidence of biological features which may be associated with personality disorders is limited. There may however be an association between impulsive or aggressive personality traits and low levels of the serotonin metabolite 5-HIAA (5-hydroxyindoleacetic acid) or high androgen levels. Dissocial personality disorder may be associated with EEG abnormalities.

Epidemiology
There is no consensus as to the overall prevalence of personality disorders in the general population. Most estimates fall between 6% and 10%, with some studies suggesting higher rates. The lifetime prevalence, sex distribution, and associations of individual personality disorders are shown in Fig. 23.2.

Course and prognosis
Once the personality is formed by early adulthood, any traits and disorders may be assumed to remain a consistent force, influencing behaviour for a lifetime. However, some longitudinal studies of subjects with certain personality traits have shown that behaviour patterns can eventually change. This may be due to changes in life situation and circumstance—the distrust and suspicion of the paranoid patient may, for instance, diminish, and ability to sustain relationships improve. Dissocial personality disorder is the most likely to persist unmodified for a lifetime.

Many personality disorders are associated with development of depression (see Fig. 23.2). A proportion of individuals with schizoid personality disorder may progress to schizophrenia; likewise, a smaller minority of individuals with paranoid and anankastic personality disorders suffer the same fate.

Treatment
A diagnosis of personality disorder reflects that an individual has deviant aspects of behaviour and of

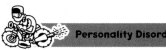

Summary of personality disorders

DSM-IV name	ICD-10 name	Striking features
paranoid PD	paranoid PD	suspicious unable to trust sensitive to setbacks
schizoid PD	schizoid PD	prefers solitude to making friends introspective and emotionally cold indifferent to praise or criticism
schizotypal PD	(listed as schizotypal disorder)	odd beliefs, thoughts or speech illusions or unusual perceptions eccentricity and lack of friends
antisocial PD	dissocial PD	no concern for others' feelings lacks guilt and blames others cannot sustain relationships
borderline PD	emotionally unstable PD borderline type (impulsive type is also listed)	uncertain self image relationships unstable dread of abandonment threatens or performs self-harm
histrionic PD	histrionic PD	self dramatises easily suggestible inappropriate seductiveness but sexually frigid
obsessive-compulsive PD	anankastic PD	perfectionism preoccupation with detail inflexibility
avoidant PD	anxious (avoidant) PD	limited by fear of rejection apprehensive feels inept but longs to be liked
dependent PD	dependent PD	depends on others/subordinates self lets others make decisions fears loneliness/abandonment
narcissistic PD	(not listed in ICD-10)	grandiose behaviour or fantasies no empathy, assumes others envious appears haughty, courts admiration

Fig. 23.1 Summary of personality disorders.

inner experience, but is not indicative of a mental illness per se. Some psychiatrists consider that personality disorders are not amenable to psychiatric treatment and do not routinely admit individuals with these disorders to the inpatient unit unless there are comorbid psychiatric disorders. Evidence of such comorbid conditions (e.g. depression, schizophrenia, anxiety and somatoform disorders) should be sought and the illnesses treated appropriately.

At best, treatment of personality disorders is slow. As changes in circumstances may moderate behaviour in patients with personality disorders,

assisting individuals in finding an appropriate lifestyle may be more helpful than attempting to radically alter personality. Given a suitable life situation, dysfunctional personality traits may produce behaviour with fewer adverse effects.

Drug treatments (Fig. 23.3) may be of some value in the short term to combat affects and emotional states engendered, but generally there is little or no long-lasting impact on the personality.

Dependent and obsessive–compulsive (anankastic) personality disorders are the most amenable to psychotherapy. Therapists need to set strict limits on what constitutes acceptable behaviour, and the initial therapeutic contract may specify an aim of working on a particular cognition or behaviour rather than hoping to effect wholesale changes to personality in the limited time of therapy.

Prevalence, sex distribution, and associations of personality disorders			
Personality disorder	**Prevalence**	**Male:Female**	**Associations**
paranoid	0.5–2.5%	m>f	schizophrenia
schizoid	up to 7%	2:1	schizophrenia
schizotypal	3%	unknown	schizophrenia
dissocial	2%	3:1	alcohol and substance misuse, paraphilias
borderline	1–2%	1:2	depression/bipolar disorder
histrionic	2–3%	f > >m	depression; somatization disorder
obsessive-compulsive/ anankastic	unknown	m > f	depression, schizophrenia
avoidant/anxious	1–10%	unknown	generalized anxiety disorder, depression
dependant	unknown	f > m	depression
narcissistic	<1 %	m >f	depression

Fig. 23.2 Prevalence, sex distribution, and associations of personality disorders.

Examples of symptoms and emotional states occurring in personality disorders which may be treated with psychotropic drugs		
Indication	**Drug**	**Personality disorders in which indication may arise**
anxiety symptoms	benzodiazepines other anxiolytics antipsychotics (if severe)	most personality disorders
autonomic symptoms	beta blockers	avoidant
control of anger	antipsychotics	borderline
ideas of reference	antipsychotics	schizotypal
low mood	antidepressants	most personality disorders

Fig. 23.3 Examples of symptoms and emotional states occurring in personality disorders which may be treated with psychotropic drugs.

Although the drugs listed in Fig. 23.3 may provide short-term relief for the symptoms or emotional states described, and may effectively treat comorbid psychiatric illnesses such as depression, remember that drug therapy is unlikely to have any long-term effect on the underlying dysfunctional personality traits.

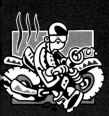

24. Child and Adolescent Psychiatry

A wide range of disorders presenting in childhood and adolescence were introduced in Chapter 11. This chapter aims to provide further information on the main categories described and an overview of treatments used. The relevant issue of child abuse and its psychiatric consequences are also included.

Patients with learning disabilities are generally managed by consultants with a special interest in learning disability; the disorders are included in this chapter because of their presentation in childhood.

THE DISORDERS OF CHILDHOOD AND ADOLESCENCE

Specific diagnostic categories

The disorders specific to childhood are summarized in Figs 24.1–24.6.

Other disorders

Elective mutism

Elective mutism is rare (<1% of child psychiatry presentations) and usually occurs in middle childhood (5–10 years). Girls are affected more than boys.

It is associated with a history of trauma, parental psychiatric illness, and a different first-language between parent(s) and child.

Enuresis

The incidence of secondary enuresis (developing after continence is established) peaks between 5–8 years, declining with age. Boys are affected more than girls; the incidence at 5 years is 7% and 3% respectively.

It is associated with delayed toilet-training, psychosocial stress, large families, lower social class, institutionalization, and a family history of enuresis.

Approximately 20% have another psychiatric problem, such as emotional disorder, night terrors, or encopresis.

Encopresis

Approximately 1% of 5-year-olds have encopresis, boys more than girls.

It also is associated with psychosocial stress and emotional disturbance.

Learning disability (mental retardation)	
aetiological theories	traditionally divided into subcultural (environmental) and pathological (organic) causation. Specific organic causes are more readily identified as the disability becomes more severe. An organic cause is not identified in ~40% of total (idiopathic). Specific causes of learning disability are shown in Fig. 24.2
epidemiology	prevalence: <2% (85% mild, 10% moderate, 4% severe, 1% profound) male>female 1.5:1 mild mental retardation is over-represented among lower socio-economic classes
investigations	diagnosis clarified by psychometric testing, e.g. British Ability Scores, Wechsler Intelligence Scales For Children. Specific causes excluded by careful physical examination and relevant investigations, e.g. chromosomal studies, amino acid studies, CT scan. Both approaches are done in conjunction with clinical/educational psychologists and paediatricians
psychiatric complications	not associated with increased risk of suicide, BUT more likely to suffer from other mental disorders prevalence amongst learning disabled: • dementia ~3% (20-64 yrs), ~22% (>64 yrs) Down syndrome closely associated with Alzheimer's disease • schizophrenia ~3% • affective disorders 10-15% • obsessive compulsive disorder ~4% • personality/behavioural disorder 25-30%

Fig. 24.1 Learning disability (mental retardation).

Child abuse

Child and adolescent psychiatrists have an important role in the assessment of known or suspected cases of child abuse—usually in liaison with other professionals such as paediatricians or social workers. In addition, they may be able to provide treatments for the psychiatric problems that result.

Child abuse refers to harmful treatment of a child by an adult, either through deliberate action or neglect of the child's needs, which is unacceptable within the society they live.

Three forms are recognized:
- Physical abuse (non-accidental injury, NAI).
- Sexual abuse.
- Emotional abuse (neglect).

Physical abuse (non-accidental injury, NAI)

Physical abuse commonly presents to paediatricians or A&E departments with recurrent bruising, cuts, scolds, fractures, and poisoning. The child may present to psychiatrists with anhedonia, hypervigilance, social withdrawal, or conduct problems.

Sexual abuse

Studies suggest that around 5–10% of all under-16s suffer some form of sexual abuse, with approximately 0.5% experiencing non-consenting intercourse. Again, children may present with a variety of emotional and conduct problems (including full-blown post-traumatic stress disorder). Inappropriate sexual behaviour and curiosity beyond normal experimentation is an important warning sign.

Classifying causes of learning disability	
genetic	e.g. trisomy 21 (Down syndrome) Klinefelter syndrome (XXY), fragile X syndrome, phenlyketonuria, tuberose sclerosis
intrauterine environment	e.g. foetal alcohol syndrome, rubella infection, phenytoin exposure
pregnancy/ perinatal	e.g. low birth weight, foetal distress, neonatal infections
general medical	e.g. meningitis/encephalitis, trauma (particularly physical abuse), toxins (e.g. lead), severe epilepsy
environmental	e.g. malnutrition, socio-economic deprivation, emotional abuse

Fig. 24.2 Classification of causes of learning disability.

Fig. 24.3 Autism.

Autism	
aetiology	twin and family studies suggest a genetic component. Association with pregnancy/perinatal complications and organic causes of learning disability (Fig. 24.2)
epidemiology	prevalence ~1 per 2500 male>female 4:1 no social class difference
investigations	none specific, diagnosis clinical although clarified by IQ assessment. Increased rate of neurological 'soft' signs on examination
complications	~25% develop epilepsy often develop depression in later life
prognosis	continuous course, majority unable to work or live independently, requiring long-term care

Fig. 24.4 Hyperkinetic disorder.

Hyperkinetic disorder	
aetiology	probably mixture of constitutional (increased in first degree relatives), medical (may follow encephalitis) and environmental (e.g. child abuse) factors
epidemiology	prevalence varies between different countries, e.g. USA (5%)>UK(1%), probably as a result of different diagnostic practices male>female 9:1
investigations	no specific diagnostic tests although reported increase in minor physical abnormalities
prognosis	a minority have persistent problems into adulthood

Fig. 24.5 Conduct disorder and emotional disorders.

Conduct disorder and emotional disorders		
	Conduct disorders	**Emotional disorders**
aetiology	adoption studies suggest a genetic contribution. Particularly associated with epilepsy, global/specific learning disability and hyperkinetic syndrome. Important environmental contribution: deprivation, abuse, large families	the specific emotional disorders of childhood are thought to have a combination of genetic and environmental causes. Refer to Chapters 20–21 for aetiology of other affective/neurotic disorders
epidemiology	prevalence 4–10% adolescents urban>rural male>female ~3:1	prevalence (all emotional disorders): ~2.5% female>male ~1.5:1
prognosis	increased risk of adult dissocial personality disorder, substance use disorders and affective disorders	the specific emotional disorders of childhood do not usually persist into adulthood; more severe disorders, e.g. depressive disorder/OCD have a worse prognosis

Fig. 24.6 Tic disorders: Gilles de la Tourette's syndrome.

Tic disorders: Tourette's syndrome	
aetiology	apparent autosomal dominant pattern of inheritance, penetrance higher in females (10% show no familial pattern). Postulated dopamine (neurotransmitter) mechanism
epidemiology	prevalence ~ 1 per 2500 males>females ~ 3:1 median age of onset = 7 years
investigations	no specific diagnostic tests although other neurological conditions should be excluded. Associated with epilepsy and learning disability
complications	direct injuries from tics: retinal detachment, orthopaedic problems, skin lesions
prognosis	severe forms of Tourette's syndrome usually persist into adulthood

Munchausen's-syndrome-by-proxy is a recently described disorder whereby the parent or carer repeatedly induces or fabricates symptoms in their child in order to gain unnecessary medical treatment or investigations. Examples include administration of insulin or poisons.

Emotional abuse (neglect)

Emotional abuse is often more difficult to prove and requires careful consideration of what one would expect are a child's physical, nutritional, medical, and emotional needs. The children often present at a young age with failure to thrive or developmental delay. In later childhood, they may present with a variety of emotional and behavioural problems.

Risk factors for child abuse

These include:

- Socioeconomic deprivation.
- Large families.
- Previously abused parents/carers.
- A step-parent.
- Young, immature parents.
- Parental psychiatric illness, especially psychosis, severe affective disorders, substance misuse, and personality disorder.
- Parental criminality.
- Neonatal problems, deformity, or illness affecting the child.

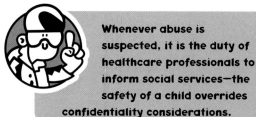 **Whenever abuse is suspected, it is the duty of healthcare professionals to inform social services—the safety of a child overrides confidentiality considerations.**

Management strategies

This section will highlight the main pharmacological and psychotherapeutic approaches to treatment in child and adolescent psychiatry.

Pharmacotherapy

Pharmacological approaches are used less frequently in this age group and often as an adjunct to a psychotherapeutic approach. Specific examples are described below.

Antipsychotics

Antipsychotics may be used for treating psychotic disorders; well-established drugs such as chlorpromazine and haloperidol tend to be favoured. They are sometimes used as an adjunct to treatment of severe behavioural disturbance, particularly in the learning-disabled. Low-dose haloperidol can be used to treat severe tic disorders.

CNS stimulants

The amphetamine analogue methylphenidate (Ritalin) is an effective treatment of hyperkinetic disorder through its enhancement of selective attention and vigilance. Side effects include headache, insomnia, growth retardation, loss of appetite, and, occasionally, tics or psychosis.

Antidepressants

Few studies have demonstrated the efficacy of treating childhood depression with antidepressants. The older tricyclic agents with a strong anticholinergic effect (e.g. imipramine) have a well-established role in the treatment of nocturnal enuresis.

Psychotherapy

Psychotherapy is usually the first-line approach to the majority of behavioural, conduct, and emotional disorders. Both psychodynamic and cognitive–behavioural forms are used, in a variety of individual and group settings.

Cognitive–behavioural methods are increasingly used for the treatment of affective disorders (e.g. depressive disorders), neurotic disorders (e.g. obsessive–compulsive disorder, phobic disorders), and behavioural disorders (e.g. enuresis, bulimia nervosa). Behavioural methods are particularly well established in the treatment of nocturnal enuresis, parents are advised to avoid criticism and positively reinforce when the child is dry (Star Charts are sometimes used to help reinforcement). Enuresis alarms, most notably the 'pad and bell' awake the child as voiding begins.

Play therapy, art therapy, and dramatherapy are particularly important for younger children who are too immature to express their feelings verbally, or older children who have difficulties engaging verbally (e.g. elective mutism).

Family therapy has developed as a distinct approach to treating a variety of childhood disorders over the last 40 years. Whole families are seen together with one or more therapists. The 'problem' or 'symptom' is viewed as an adaptive response to the specific system of family interrelationships. Depending on the approach used, the therapist or therapists then suggest interventions which the family can implement.

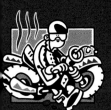

25. Psychiatry of Old Age

OLD-AGE PSYCHIATRY

Old-age psychiatry achieved recognition as a subspecialty as recently as 1989. Usually patients come under the realm of the old-age psychiatrists at the age of 65 years, but in some services the cut-off is later.

Approximately 16% of the British population is aged 65 years or over, and as life-expectancy continues to increase, this percentage is likely to rise. Life-expectancy for a 65-year-old man is now 15 years, and for a women, 20 years, and women are three times as likely as men to reach their 85th birthday.

Ageing is associated with numerous biological, social, and psychological changes.

Biological changes associated with old age include cellular and organ-system changes.

Cellular changes comprise:
- Degeneration of cells and failure of replication by cell division.
- Alteration in enzyme activity and metabolism.
- Changes in receptor sensitivity.
- Increased production of connective tissue.

Organ-system changes comprise:
- Enlargement of the heart and increased vascular resistance.
- Reduction in lung capacity.
- Decreased blood flow to the cerebrum, kidneys, liver, and bowel.
- Loss of acuity in all senses (e.g. lens thickening).
- Degeneration of bone, leading to osteoporosis and fragility.
- Prostatic enlargement.
- Altered hormone production (e.g. reduction in sex hormone levels).

The above changes may produce subtle alterations in function which may be regarded as 'normal for old age'. More significant biological alterations produce disease (Fig. 25.1).

Social and psychological challenges include:
- Retirement.
- Deteriorating financial position.
- Geographical separation from family.
- Bereavement of spouse or of contemporaries.
- Reduced sexual activity.
- Coping with illness, disability, and approaching death.

The old-age psychiatry service
Old-age psychiatrists and their multidisciplinary team see patients in:
- Domicilliary visits at the patient's residence (own home, relative's home, or nursing or residential home).
- Outpatient clinics.

Prevalence of common general medical conditions and syndromes in the elderly	
Condition or syndrome	Prevalence in elderly (%)
osteo or rheumatoid arthritis	50
hypertension	35
ischaemic heart disease	25
diabetes	9
deafness/ partial deafness	28
blindness	9

Fig. 25.1 Prevalence of common general medical conditions and syndromes in the elderly.

- Day hospitals.
- Inpatient wards.

As the needs and prognosis of patients with dementia may be very different to those of elderly patients with other mental illnesses, separate inpatient wards are usually provided for 'organic' (dementia and confusional states) and 'functional' (most other disorders including mood disorders and schizophrenia) groups.

Admission to an inpatient bed may be indicated for:
- Assessment and treatment of functional disorders.
- Risk management of a suicidal or dangerous patient.
- Assessment of the mental state and functioning of a patient showing signs of early dementia (assessment may be performed in outpatients or the day hospital, but services may provide specific assessment beds allowing patients to be monitored intensively for 2–3 weeks before recommendations are made on support required or placement in residential or nursing care).
- Emergency admission due to acute exacerbations of symptoms in patients with functional or organic disorders.
- Planned admissions for rehabilitation and to allow respite for carers of patients with organic disorders.

An old-age psychiatry team will include consultant and trainee psychiatrists, ward-based and community psychiatric nurses, social workers, an occupational therapist, and a pharmacist. There should be access to physiotherapy, psychology, and speech therapy services, and close liaison with physicians specializing in elderly medicine.

Epidemiology of mental illness in the elderly

The most prevalent psychiatric diagnoses in the elderly population are:
- Dementia.
- Depression.
- Alcohol and substance-related disorders.

Dementia

Moderate or severe dementia affects 5% of those aged 65 and over and becomes more common with increasing age, affecting 10% of those aged 75 or more and 20% of those aged 85 and over. In the majority, the dementia is secondary to Alzheimer's disease—mean life-expectancy from onset being 7 years. Multi-infarct dementia has a slightly worse prognosis as affected patients are inevitably at a significant risk of death through myocardial infarction and further cerebrovascular accidents.

An assessment admission for an elderly person with suspected symptoms of dementia should include:
- Confirming the diagnosis through history, mental state examination, further tests of cognitive functioning, and liaison with relatives or carers.
- Exclusion of a potentially treatable physical cause for dementia (see Chapter 6) by physical examination and laboratory tests.
- In patients who appear depressed, exclusion of 'pseudodementia' (i.e. cognitive impairment secondary to severe depression which resolves on antidepressant treatment).
- Assessing the ability to function in the light of the clinical features present, and the need for social services support or residential placement. This usually necessitates a visit to the patient's home.

Depressive disorders

Although the peak ages for a first onset of depression occur much earlier, depression is common in the elderly, with as many as 10% having depressive symptoms at any one time. Those who first experience the illness after the age of 65 are prone to have recurrent episodes. Rates are higher in residential homes, and among the widowed and those with chronic medical problems. The elderly depressed tend to have more somatic symptoms, and features such as agitation, poor self-esteem, and paranoid ideas are common.

Suicidal ideation is also common in elderly depressed patients. Although parasuicide is less common in the elderly than in other age groups, the risk of completed suicide increases markedly with age.

Alcohol and substance use

Alcohol abuse is less prevalent in the elderly than in younger age groups. Some elderly alcoholics have a history of excess consumption since early adulthood, but others began drinking excessively to cope with the many stresses of old age. Alcohol problems are most common in the widowed and divorced and are associated with the presence of other mental and physical illnesses that may provoke (e.g. anxiety disorders) or be a consequence of (Wernicke–Korsakoff syndrome) excess consumption.

Dependence on benzodiazepines and other anxiolytics or hypnotics is common in the over-65s. Other drugs that may be 'abused' are opiates, other analgaesics (including over-the-counter preparations), and laxatives.

Other psychiatric disorders

Anxiety disorders usually have their onset earlier in life, but many elderly patients continue to suffer from previously established conditions. Specific phobia is a notable exception, as a first episode often occurs after the age of 65.

Schizophrenia most often presents in the second or third decade of life, but there is a late-onset variant (paraphrenia) which may present in old age. Note that approximately one-fifth of schizophrenics whose illness began in their youth show no symptoms by the age of 65.

Sleep problems of all types (see Chapter 22) are especially common in old age. Sleep architecture tends to change with age: total REM (rapid eye movement) sleep and stages III and IV diminish, with an increase in stages I and II. Early morning wakening is a characteristic problem in the elderly.

Interviewing the elderly patient

When interviewing elderly patients, meaningful points to consider are:
- Establishing rapport is as important as ever; some old people expect a doctor or medical student to act in a formal manner, e.g. to address the patient by their title and surname.
- Elderly patients may be slower to respond; minor memory lapses are the norm.
- The interview may be made more difficult if the patient has sensory deficits, especially deafness, or difficulties in concentration or comprehension. The interviewer needs to accommodate such problems by clarity and persistence in questioning.
- The extent of symptoms may be played down. Closed questions may be needed to overcome this problem.
- Medical students and younger doctors may be

reluctant to broach subjects such as sexual history. Such inhibitions should be overcome—the elderly are generally as willing as any age group to discuss sexual history, and an alteration in sexual behaviour may be very relevant to the case.

Other important aspects of history are:
- Past medical history—concurrent medical illness is common and may influence onset of psychiatric symptoms.
- Drug history—many elderly patients are on a variety of drugs for medical complaints.
- Family history (e.g. depression, Alzheimer's disease, other dementia).
- Marital history and details of grief for spouse if bereaved.
- Details of residence, carers, support required, and input from social services.

The mental state examination is conducted as in the general section, but a greater emphasis is placed on language and cognitive function—in particular, tests of memory, concentration, reading, writing, and intellectual tasks.

Remember that a failure in a cognitive test in the mental state examination may represent one of several deficits: for example, failure to respond to a question on the name of the hospital may reflect disorientation in place, memory loss, poor attention or concentration, dysphasia, hearing problems, or poor motivation.

Mental state examination not only provides diagnostic information but can also be used to monitor progress and variation in a patient's cognitive abilities. Many units employ a standard rating scale such as Folstein's Mini-Mental State Exam, in which a patient's score (from 0 to 30) may be monitored over time.

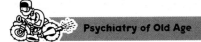

It may be useful—and with a cognitively impaired patient, essential—to obtain a collateral history from a relative or neighbour who can provide information on premorbid level of functioning and the time-course of impairment.

Pharmacology and other treatment

Drug therapy is widely used for mental health problems in the elderly, especially in functional disorders. All drug classes used in general psychiatry may be used in the elderly, but the prescriber must be mindful of the potential ramifications the cellular and bodily changes of advancing age may have on drug action. For example:

- Owing to changes in liver and renal function, drug kinetics are altered. Much lower doses may be needed to achieve a response, but side effects may also occur at a lesser dose level. It is generally advisable to use a lower starting dose and titrate up gradually, being vigilant for the onset of adverse effects. For example, the elderly are prone to postural hypotension with tricyclic antidepressants and to extrapyramidal side effects with antipsychotics.
- As many elderly people have concurrent medical illnesses (see Fig. 25.1), they tend to use more medications than the general population. Given the above pharmacokinetic changes, the potential for interactions may be greatly increased.
- Complicated regimens or impaired understanding may lead to poor compliance with treatment.

When psychotherapy is used in old-age psychiatry, it is usually undertaken on a time-limited basis (as opposed to open-ended therapies) to help the person overcome current problems. Patients with dementia may benefit from exercises such as reminiscence, in which cues from earlier in life—such as photographs of film stars of the past or songs from World War II—are used to stimulate remote memory.

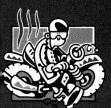

26. Forensic Psychiatry

FORENSIC PSYCHIATRY

Most medical students obtain some experience of this large subspeciality within psychiatry. This chapter provides a brief overview of this subject, with particular emphasis on areas that overlap with general psychiatry.

Forensic psychiatry is involved with:

- Assessment and management of mentally abnormal offenders; this involves close liaison with the legal system.
- Liaison with general psychiatrists over the assessment and management of potentially dangerous and severely disturbed patients.

The psychopathology associated with this speciality is much the same as it is in general adult psychiatry, although there is a greater representation of psychotic disorders (schizophrenia, severe affective disorders), substance-misuse, and personality disorders.

Historical aspects

Although forensic psychiatry is a relatively new speciality—largely developed in the last 30 years—there is a long history of mentally abnormal offenders receiving different management to other offenders by the legal system.

Important landmarks are as follows:

- The Criminal Lunatics Act 1800 first recognized that a person may be unfit to plead at the time of a trial. Fitness to plead remains an important part of assessment and depends on the ability of defendants to understand the charge, understand the effects of a plea, understand the evidence, challenge a juror, and instruct a lawyer. Defendants with dementia, learning disability, or psychotic disorders are most likely to be unfit to plead.
- In 1843, Daniel McNaughton killed a government official as a result of a long-standing paranoid delusional system: he was found not guilty on the grounds of insanity and committed to Bethlem Hospital.

The 'McNaughton Rules' established the plea 'not guilty by reasons of insanity', although this defence was largely superseded by the Homicide Act 1957.

- The Infanticide Act 1922 defined infanticide as the killing of a child by its mother in the first 12 months of life when the 'balance of her mind was disturbed' as a result of the effects of childbirth or lactation.
- The Homicide Act 1957 introduced the term 'diminished responsibility' for killings where the defendant was suffering from 'an abnormality of mind...as substantially impaired his mental responsibility'. Section 2: manslaughter (as it is otherwise known) usually leads to secure-hospital treatment when the defendant has a mental disorder.
- Part III of the Mental Health Act 1983 deals with mentally disordered individuals who are involved in criminal proceedings. It has provisions for assessment and treatment of defendants awaiting trial or sentence, treatment of convicted offenders after sentence, and transfer of prisoners to secure hospitals.

For example, a Section 37 hospital order is imposed by courts (following medical recommendations) to direct mentally disordered offenders to hospital for treatment—in practice it is almost exactly the same as a Section 3. For more serious and persistent offenders, the judge can impose, in addition, a Section 41 or 49 restriction order. This means only the Home Office can grant leave or discharge from hospital; therefore, a patient detained under Section 37/41 (both Sections are recorded) cannot be discharged by the consultant alone.

Service provision

The management of offenders who are mentally disordered or of general psychiatric patients who are a risk to others often requires treatment and rehabilitation in a secure environment. Deciding on the level of security required is an important role of the forensic psychiatrist; the following headings outline the main areas of service provision.

Special hospitals

Broadmoor, Rampton, Ashworth, and Carstairs Hospitals provide conditions of high security for approximately 1500 patients. They provide long-stay (~7 years average) facilities for patients considered to be at a 'grave immediate danger to the public'. The future of these large institutions is uncertain: many of those patients considered to be at less risk to the public have already moved to conditions of lesser security.

Regional secure units

Regional secure units are smaller (<100 beds each) and provide conditions of medium security for patients within each health region of England and Wales. They have developed in the last 20 years and are likely to increase secure provision as the special hospitals reduce capacity; the average length of stay in these units is shorter (~2 years).

Low-security provision

A variety of small low-security units exist across the country (often a locked ward within the main hospital), largely providing short-term management of patients too disturbed for general wards. They have a smaller proportion of Part III patients than the above.

Community services

Many psychiatric services have now developed closer links with local courts (court diversion schemes) and probation services, to provide earlier recognition and treatment of mentally disordered offenders. Most forensic psychiatrists have regular clinics at local prisons. The scale of mental disorder within prisons is much higher than in the general population: a recent survey of remand prisoners (pretrial) showed a 63% prevalence of mental disorder—11% were psychotic.

Crime and mental disorder

Most convicted criminals do not have a mental disorder and most mentally disordered do not break the law. The strongest predictors of criminal activity in general, are sociological: young, unemployed, urban men. Attempts to establish a relationship between mental disorder and crime are hampered by a number of factors, e.g. inaccuracy of actual crime figures and 'diversion' of

mentally disordered offenders to hospital without a conviction recorded.

The findings for specific diagnostic categories are summarized below.

Disorders related to substance misuse

Substance-misuse disorders were the largest diagnostic group in a recent survey of mentally disordered remand prisoners. The association between alcohol and violent crime, and between the use of illegal substances and acquisitive offences, is detailed in Chapter 18. Again, this relationship may in fact be more due to sociological and personal factors than to direct causation.

Schizophrenia

The link between schizophrenia and violence continues to receive considerable media attention spotlighting alleged failures of community care. There is no evidence of increasing homicides by schizophrenic patients in the last 30 years, nor do this group have a higher rate of offending than the general population. However, there is evidence that schizophrenic patients commit a higher proportion of violent offences than the general population and this is often related to positive symptoms (delusions, hallucinations).

Affective disorders

Mania/hypomania is associated with increased offending behaviour; this is related to both the effects of overarousal (overactivity, sexual disinhibition, aggression) and the effects of paranoid delusions or hallucinations. The association with violence is not as strong as for schizophrenia. Non-psychotic depressive disorders appear to be particularly linked to shoplifting, whereas severe psychotic depression with delusions of guilt, persecution, unworthiness, and jealousy may lead to crimes of violence before suicide.

Personality disorders

Within prison and secure-hospital populations, there are high rates of personality disorder— especially dissocial, paranoid, and borderline forms. Dissocial personality disorder, in particular, is associated with crime and has been diagnosed in around 20% of prisoners; the picture is often complicated by comorbid substance misuse.

Psychopathic disorder is a legal definition defined in Section I of the Mental Health Act 1983 (see Chapter 16) rather than a medical classification of personality disorder. To be detained under this category, the patient must be considered treatable. Despite the difficulty establishing treatability, approximately 25% of special-hospital patients are detained under this category.

Learning disability

People with learning disability are more likely to be convicted of criminal offences in general; this seems to be due to a number of factors, e.g. more easily caught, easily exploited by others. Compared with the general population, they are over-represented in convictions for sex offences and arson.

Dangerousness

Recent media interest into violence and homicides committed by the mentally disordered has increased expectations on mental health services to predict the risk of dangerous behaviour. The proportion of homicides by the mentally disordered is around 10%—this proportion is falling because of the general increase in all homicides. Of the mentally disordered, around half will have had contact with mental health services in the year before the offence. Whether more careful risk assessment could reduce these figures and those for violent offences in general among the mentally disordered is uncertain: conventional wisdom suggests psychiatrists are too cautious, with only one-third of those predicted to be dangerous actually proving to be so.

Like suicide prediction, prediction of dangerousness assumes risk is not static and will vary according to changes in mental state and social context—usually, only immediate or short-term risk can be commented on.

The factors in a patient's history and mental state relevant to assessment of dangerousness are listed in Fig. 26.1.

Risk factors for dangerousness

History
- previous violence (the most important predictor of future violence)
- substance misuse
- poor compliance with psychiatric care, and recent discontinuation of treatment
- recent severe stress
- 'rootlessness'—disorganized relationships, unstable employment and living conditions
- access to potential victims or weapons

Mental state
- behaviour—agitation, irritability, hostility, suspiciousness
- mood—anger, e.g. is the patient making specific threats and what does he intend to do?
- thoughts—persecutory delusions, delusions of jealousy, delusions of passivity
- perceptions—derogatory or command auditory hallucinations

Fig. 26.1 Risk factors for dangerousness.

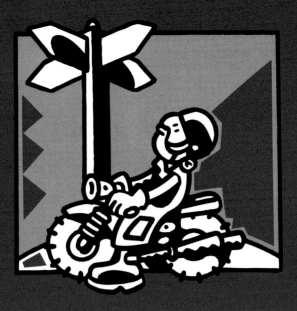

SELF-ASSESSMENT

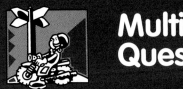

Multiple-choice Questions

Indicate whether each answer is true or false.

1. Delusional ideas:

a) Are a symptom of psychosis.
b) Are characteristic of personality disorder.
c) Are always false.
d) Are easily understood within a person's cultural background.
e) Are characteristic of anorexia nervosa.

2. Hallucinations:

a) May occur in a normal bereavement reaction.
b) On waking from sleep are termed hypnagogic.
c) Are frequently misinterpretations of external stimuli.
d) May be shared by a close relative in 'folie á deux'.
e) Are a characteristic symptom of paranoid schizophrenia.

3. Schizophrenia:

a) Has a peak age of onset for females at 15–25 years.
b) Is more common in men.
c) Has been related to limbic dopamine depletion.
d) Has a higher incidence in higher social classes.
e) Was first described by Schneider.

4. Regular use of amphetamine:

a) Can lead to tolerance.
b) Can be stopped abruptly without serious physical consequences.
c) Invariably causes psychosis.
d) May cause dementia.
e) Is often associated with weight gain.

5. Delirium tremens:

a) Can be managed in the community.
b) Is characterized by Lilliputian hallucinations.
c) Usually occurs within 5 days of cessation of drinking.
d) Is associated with tachycardia and pupil dilatation.
e) Is primarily treated by an antipsychotic drug.

6. The following are correctly paired:

a) Autism and psychosis.
b) Freud and cognitive behavioural therapy.
c) Alzheimer's disease and neurofibrillary tangles.
d) Delirium and impaired short-term memory.
e) Schizophrenia and neologisms.

7. A 55-year-old man scores 25/30 on the Mini-Mental State Examination; his performance could be explained by:

a) Generalized anxiety.
b) Normal age-related cognitive decline.
c) A dissociative disorder.
d) A depressive disorder.
e) An anankastic personality disorder.

8. The following are forms of thought-disorder:

a) Word salad.
b) Pressure of speech.
c) Thought-echo.
d) Flight of ideas.
e) Waxy flexibility.

9. Regarding dementia:

a) Creutzfeldt–Jakob disease is a form of spongiform encephalopathy.
b) Diffuse Lewy body disease has a better prognosis than Alzheimer's disease.
c) HIV dementia occurs in about 50% of AIDS cases.
d) Huntington's disease is caused by a variable number triple repeat on chromosome 6.
e) Pick's disease is characterized by atrophy of frontal and temporal lobes.

10. Regarding patients with learning disability:

a) They have a higher rate of suicide.
b) They have a higher rate of schizophrenia.
c) The prevalence is higher in males.
d) They have the childhood equivalent of dementia.
e) Most mild forms have a recognized physical cause.

11. The Mental Health Act 1983:

a) Authorizes emergency treatment of unconscious patients.
b) Allows compulsory treatment under Section 2.
c) Allows a doctor to instigate a Section 5(4) holding order.
d) Does not define mental illness.
e) Does not authorize compulsory drug treatment outside hospital.

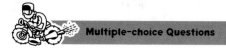

12. The following are associated with dissocial personality disorder:

a) Increased risk of violent crime.
b) Former childhood conduct disorder.
c) Excessive guilt for consequences of behaviour.
d) Increased risk of suicide.
e) Often successful personal functioning.

13. Puerperal psychosis:

a) Occurs after 1% of pregnancies.
b) Is characterized by persistent delusions and hallucinations.
c) Is caused by changing oestrogen levels after birth.
d) Has the same incidence irrespective of a woman's past psychiatric history.
e) May be associated with clouding of consciousness.

14. The following are correctly paired:

a) Fetishism and sexual arousal through inanimate objects.
b) Transsexualism and sexual arousal through wearing opposite-sex clothing.
c) Delayed ejaculation and fluoxetine.
d) Premature ejaculation and spinal cord injury.
e) Dysfunctional sexual desire and hyperprolactinaemia.

15. Regarding disorders of childhood:

a) Coprolalia is pathognomonic of Tourette's syndrome.
b) Hyperkinetic disorder should be treated with antipsychotics.
c) Family therapy is used in the treatment of conduct disorder.
d) Encopresis is considered normal at 6 years.
e) Children with elective mutism usually have normal premorbid language development.

16. Complications of excessive alcohol consumption include:

a) Hypomagnesaemia.
b) Amnesic syndrome.
c) Psychotic symptoms.
d) Macrocytosis.
e) Increased vulnerability to violent crime.

17. Head injury may cause:

a) Delirium.
b) Affective psychosis.
c) Pick's disease.
d) Organic personality disorder.
e) Insomnia.

18. The following are characteristic of schizophrenia:

a) Flight of ideas.
b) Derailment.
c) Delusions of control.
d) Self-mutilation.
e) Hearing thoughts spoken aloud.

19. The following increase the risk of violence:

a) Delusions of jealousy.
b) Command hallucinations urging the subject to kill.
c) Psychomotor retardation.
d) History of violent convictions.
e) Obsessional thoughts of violence.

20. In the treatment of substance dependence:

a) Disulfiram enhances GABA transmission.
b) Lofexidine is an α-adrenoreceptor agonist.
c) Methadone is preferable to heroin because of its increased safety in overdose.
d) Better results are achieved with married patients.
e) Alcohol withdrawal is facilitated with vitamin B_1 treatment.

21. The following conditions may cause an organic psychotic disorder:

a) Systemic lupus erythematosus.
b) AIDS.
c) Hypocalcaemia.
d) Hyperglycaemia.
e) Vitamin B_{12} deficiency.

22. In the cognitive assessment:

a) Asking the patient to name the Prime Minister tests episodic memory.
b) The digit span test tests short-term (primary) memory.
c) Repeating the months of the year backwards tests concentration.
d) Asking the patient to complete a three-step command tests parietal lobe function.
e) Abnormalities of motor sequencing suggest frontal lobe damage.

23. Alzheimer's disease:

a) Is more common among smokers.
b) Is sometimes treated with cholinergic drugs.
c) Can be diagnosed on CT scanning alone.
d) Develops in Down syndrome.
e) Is associated with β-amyloid deposition.

24. Regarding psychological treatments:

a) Psychodynamic therapies utilize transference relationships in the therapeutic process.
b) Desensitization is a useful treatment for phobias.
c) Cognitive techniques interpret unconscious processes.
d) Alcohol dependence is unresponsive to psychotherapy.
e) Obsessive–compulsive disorder responds better to cognitive behavioural therapy than to psychodynamic therapy.

25. The following suggest delirium:

a) Alterations in consciousness.
b) 'Belle indifference' to their problems.
c) Visual hallucinations.
d) Insidious onset of cognitive dysfunction.
e) Symptoms improving at night.

26. Biological or somatic symptoms of depression include:

a) Hypersomnia.
b) Anhedonia.
c) Hopelessness.
d) Increased appetite.
e) Loss of libido.

27. Depressive symptoms may be secondary to:

a) Anorexia nervosa.
b) Schizophrenia.
c) Alzheimer's disease.
d) Addison's disease.
e) Rheumatoid arthritis.

28. Anhedonia may occur during:

a) A depressive episode.
b) A hypomanic episode.
c) A normal bereavement reaction.
d) Dysthymia.
e) A psychotic episode.

29. The following may occur in manic episodes but not in hypomanic episodes:

a) Flight of ideas.
b) Grandiose delusions.
c) Cachexia.
d) Increased talkativeness.
e) Erratic sleep pattern.

30. Free-floating anxiety:

a) Occurs only in predictable situations such as in aeroplanes or at sea.
b) Is a characteristic feature of social phobia.
c) Is usually experienced as discrete episodes lasting 5–10 minutes.
d) Is an essential feature of generalized anxiety disorder.
e) May occur without there being an obvious external threat.

31. The following are recognized as panic attack symptoms:

a) Chest tightness.
b) Flushing.
c) Depersonalization.
d) Tinnitus.
e) Muscle tension.

32. Obsessional thoughts:

a) Are recognized by the subject as a product of his or her own mind.
b) Commonly occur in post-traumatic stress disorder.
c) Are usually seen as entirely reasonable by the patient.
d) May be accompaied by compulsive acts which heighten anxiety.
e) Are a recognized feature of histrionic personality disorder.

33. Clinical features of post-traumatic stress disorder include:

a) Avoidance.
b) Exaggerated startle response.
c) Flashbacks.
d) Hypervigilance.
e) Episodic dizziness.

34. The following statements are true:

a) Somatization disorder involves a belief of having one or more serious physical diseases.
b) Most psychiatric inpatients who experience recurrent chest pain have somatization disorder.
c) Dysmorphophobia may involve a persistent belief of having abnormal facial features.
d) Malingering is differentiated from factitious disorder by the intensity of the feigned symptoms.
e) Depressive disorders should be considered before diagnosing somatization disorder.

35. Losing weight may lead to development of:

a) Cachexia.
b) Lanugo.
c) Hypercholesterolaemia.
d) Manic episodes.
e) Amenorrhoea.

36. Patients with bulimia nervosa:

a) Must weigh considerably less than the recommended weight for their height.
b) If female, usually have amenorrhoea.
c) May take laxatives to prevent weight gain.
d) Become disinterested in food soon after onset of the illness.
e) May have hyperkalaemia as a consequence of repeated vomiting.

37. Hypersomnia may be caused by:

a) Narcolepsy.
b) Depressive disorders.
c) Treatment with SSRI antidepressants.
d) Treatment with chlorpromazine.
e) Uraemia.

38. Patients who have survived a suicide attempt:

a) Must be admitted to a psychiatric ward for further assessment.
b) Should not be asked about ongoing suicidal ideas for fear of provoking a further attempt.
c) Are more often female than male.
d) Are more likely to have engaged in substance misuse than the general population.
e) Are at increased risk of subsequent completed suicide if suffering from anorexia nervosa.

39. Catatonic features of schizophrenia include:

a) Mannerisms.
b) Third-person auditory hallicinations.
c) Stupor.
d) Passivity phenomena.
e) Stereotypies.

40. Regarding antidepressants:

a) SSRIs are more effective in treating depressive symptoms than tricyclic agents.
b) A patient prescribed lofepramine must avoid cheese, chianti wine, and yeast extracts.
c) Anticholinergic effects include nausea and headache.
d) Lithium augmentation is a standard strategy for treating schizophrenia.
e) Tricyclics are routinely combined with phenelzine to treat severe depressive episodes.

41. Clozapine:

a) Requires regular haematological monitoring in case of aplastic anaemia.
b) Causes less anticholinergic (antimuscarinic) effects than haloperidol.
c) Is less likely to cause extrapyramidal side effects than haloperidol.
d) Is as sedative as thioridazine.
e) Is more likely to be effective against negative symptoms of schizophrenia than conventional antipsychotics.

42. The following statements about drugs are true:

a) Lithium is mainly broken down by the liver.
b) Benzodiazepines exert their action by binding to the dopamine receptor.
c) Zopiclone is an alternative to temazepam for insomnia.
d) Tardive dyskinesia may be abolished by antimuscarinc drugs.
e) Antipsychotics lower the convulsion threshold.

43. The following are features of borderline personality disorder:

a) Recurrent self-harm.
b) Preoccupation with detail.
c) Unstable relationships.
d) Fear of abandoment.
e) Self-dramatization.

44. Erectile dysfunction may be caused by:

a) Diabetes mellitus.
b) Amitriptyline treatment.
c) Depressive disorders.
d) Performance anxiety.
e) Manic episodes.

45. Concerning puerperal psychosis:

a) It is more common in a first pregnancy than subsequent pregnancies.
b) It may be treated with lithium in breastfeeding patients.
c) Treatment may require separation of mother and baby.
d) Symptoms usually occur within 3 days of birth.
e) Family history of depression is a risk factor.

46. Regarding anxiety disorders:

a) Generalized anxiety disorder is more common in women than men.
b) Cognitive behavioural therapy is an effective treatment in many anxiety disorders.
c) Post-traumatic stress disorder symptoms usually begin within 2–4 weeks of exposure to a severe or catastrophic stressor.
d) Tricyclic antidepressants are as effective in generalized anxiety disorder as in panic disorder.
e) Onset of obsessive–compulsive disorder is usually between the ages of 25 and 40 years.

47. The following personality disorders are correctly paired with the psychiatric disorder with which they are associated:

a) Anankastic—depression.
b) Histrionic—somatization disorder.
c) Dependent—depression.
d) Schizoid—bipolar affective disorder.
e) Dissocial—alcohol and substance misuse.

48. The following are associated with advancing age:

a) Increased parasuicide risk.
b) Increased risk of alcohol abuse.
c) Reduction in REM sleep.
d) Worsening of symptoms in depression.
e) Increased risk of postural hypotension with tricyclic antidepressants.

49. Social phobia:

a) Predominantly affects females.
b) Has onset most commonly in the teenage years.
c) May be associated with avoidance.
d) May be secondary to depressive disorders.
e) Can be exacerbated by β-blocking drugs.

50. Drugs which often provoke withdrawal syndromes when stopped abruptly include:

a) Lorazepam.
b) Fluoxetine.
c) Lofexidine.
d) Nicotine.
e) Cannabis.

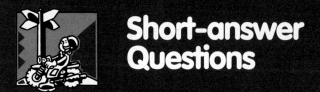

Short-answer Questions

1. What are Schneider's first-rank symptoms?

2. Name five general medical disorders that can cause psychosis.

3. What are the features of alcohol-dependence syndrome?

4. Define 'personality'. What are the diagnostic guidelines for personality disorder?

5. List ten causes of dementia.

6. What features distinguish a puerperal psychosis from a schizophrenic or affective psychosis?

7. How are the psychiatric disorders of childhood and adolescence classified?

8. What categories of mental disorder are included in the Mental Health Act 1983? How do Sections 2 and 3 differ?

9. What are the principles to the management of delirium?

10. Define formal thought-disorder. What are the commonly described abnormalities?

11. What are the three main categories of antidepressants? State three common side effects for each group.

12. What is 'free-floating anxiety'? What forms of drug therapy and psychotherapy are useful in the management of generalized anxiety disorder?

13. Describe four clinical features of borderline personality disorder. To what extent is this disorder treatable by: a) drug therapy; b) psychotherapy?

14. Define anhedonia and list five further biological (somatic) and four cognitive symptoms of depression.

15. Outline the definition of: a) obsessions; b) compulsions. List three pairs of obsessions and compulsions that often occur together.

16. What are the main differences between anorexia nervosa and bulimia nervosa? Name four other psychiatric illnesses and four physical disorders which may cause weight loss.

17. What are the key differences between: a) suicide and parasuicide; b) parasuicide and deliberate self-harm? List four psychiatric disorders that are associated with completed suicide.

18. List the three main psychiatric syndromes that are associated with the puerperium. Give their prevalences and indicate briefly how each is managed.

19. A depressed patient who had no benefit from 6 weeks' therapy with fluoxetine fails to respond to an adequate dose of a tricyclic antidepressant after a similar period of treatment. What advice should a psychiatrist who is considering lithium augmentation give the patient about the good and bad points of this treatment?

20. List ten of the recognized symptoms of panic attacks. What conditions must be satisfied to make a diagnosis of panic disorder?

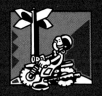

Patient Management Problems

1. A 46-year-old man tells his general practitioner that he has been feeling miserable for most of the time over the last 3 years, blaming: a) his job, which involves both driving and making important management decisions; and b) a tendency to suffer from recurrent coughs and colds, relieved only by heavy doses of cold remedies.

   - What questions should the GP ask to establish whether he has a diagnosis of (major) depression?
   - If he falls short of having depression, what criteria would he need to meet to have a diagnosis of dysthymia?
   - Describe the treatment options for dysthymia. Which antidepressants might you wish to avoid as first-line treatment given this man's history?

---

2. A 32-year-old man with a long history of mental illness describes a history of marked insomnia over the past 2 months, involving difficulty in getting to sleep, repeated awakening, and early final waking.

   - What are the possible causes of this sleep disturbance and what aspects of the history are essential to making an assessment?

---

3. A 28-year-old man has had frequent contact with psychiatric services over the past 3 years and has been diagnosed as having borderline personality disorder. He arrives at casualty at 1a.m. and asks to see a psychiatrist, insisting that if he is feeling so low that if he is not admitted he will go home and 'do away with himself'.

   - What factors are important in assessing the risk of suicide?
   - What possible courses of action might the psychiatrist recommend other than inpatient admission ?

4. A year ago, a 68-year-old lady called round to see her elder sister and was shocked to find that she had collapsed and died of what proved to be a heart attack. After initial disbelief, she became angry that she had had to be the first on the scene and had therefore been subjected to this awful finding. For a few weeks she was sad and tearful over the affair, but then seemed to put it behind her and carry on with her life as before. Two months ago she began to experience flashbacks to the event. She became reluctant to visit friends in case the same thing should happen and complained of difficulty sleeping, hypervigilance, and poor concentration.

   - How would her reaction of a year ago be described?
   - What is the likely psychiatric diagnosis at present? Justify your answer with reference to her symptoms.
   - What is the usual course and prognosis of her present problem, and how should it be managed?

---

5. A 37-year-old man with a previous history of depressive episodes for which he continues to take an antidepressant, is brought to casualty by his girlfriend. Whilst she is very concerned that he has been acting 'completely out of character' for the last few days, having apparently endless resources of energy, sleeping very little, driving his car recklessly, and spending money like never before, the patient is adamant that there is no problem and states condescendingly that he is 'insulted to be dragged along here and interrogated by the junior ranks'.

   - What is the most likely diagnosis?
   - Give a differential diagnosis and state further questions you would ask to clarify the diagnosis.
   - What alterations to his present drug treatment would be valuable if the most likely diagnosis was correct?

6. A 50-year-old woman is admitted with a first-episode psychosis characterized by third-person auditory hallucinations and delusions of grandeur.

- What is the differential diagnosis?

> As the case description is brief, use the diagnostic hierarchy to establish a wide differential.

- What physical investigations are indicated?
- Her consultant diagnoses schizophrenia. What physical, psychological, and social aspects of management should be considered?

7. A 27-year-old woman with a 6-year history of alcohol dependence is admitted for elective detoxification.

- What are the dangers of inadequately managed detoxification?
- What associated medical disorders may be detected on physical examination and investigation?
- What strategies may be used to reduce the risk of relapse after discharge?

8. You are a casualty officer asked to see a man presenting with a paracetamol overdose. He refuses blood levels and treatment. His partner believes he took approximately 50 tablets with half a bottle of whisky. His psychiatric notes reveal a history of depressive disorder with psychotic symptoms.

- What aspects of his history and mental state are helpful when predicting suicide risk?
- What legal sanctions may be used to enforce medical treatment of his overdose?
- The duty psychiatrist decides admission under the Mental Health Act is necessary. Which Sections of the Act could be used and who is required for their completion?

9. A 55-year-old man attends outpatients; his wife complains he is losing his memory.

- What is the differential diagnosis?
- How might the primary diagnosis be clarified by the history and mental state examination?

The results of his assessment suggest a presenile Alzheimer's dementia.

- What do you tell his wife about his prognosis and how would you structure management of this condition?

10. You are a casualty officer asked to see a man described as 'threatening and menacing' by the nursing staff. He was brought to the department by the police and is known to suffer from schizophrenia.

- How would you maximize your personal safety during assessment?
- What factors in the history and mental state examination are indicators of future dangerousness?

He is eventually admitted under Section 3 of the Mental Health Act for a relapse of his disorder. His psychotic symptoms are successfully treated with antipsychotic drugs, but his consultant is concerned that he is potentially dangerous during relapses.

- What long-term management options should be considered after discharge?

> Think of long-term biological, psychological, and social aspects of management, plus recent community-care health policy.

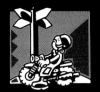
1. (a)T, (b)F, (c)F, (d)F, (e)F
2. (a)T, (b)F, (c)F, (d)F, (e)T
3. (a)F, (b)F, (c)F, (d)F, (e)F
4. (a)T, (b)T, (c)F, (d)F, (e)F
5. (a)F, (b)T, (c)T, (d)T, (e)F
6. (a)F, (b)F, (c)T, (d)T, (e)T
7. (a)T, (b)F, (c)T, (d)T, (e)F
8. (a)T, (b)F, (c)F, (d)T, (e)F
9. (a)T, (b)F, (c)T, (d)F, (e)T
10. (a)F, (b)T, (c)T, (d)F, (e)F
11. (a)F, (b)T, (c)F, (d)T, (e)T
12. (a)T, (b)T, (c)F, (d)T, (e)F
13. (a)F, (b)F, (c)F, (d)F, (e)T
14. (a)T, (b)F, (c)T, (d)F, (e)T
15. (a)F, (b)F, (c)T, (d)F, (e)T
16. (a)T, (b)T, (c)T, (d)T, (e)T
17. (a)T, (b)T, (c)F, (d)T, (e)T
18. (a)F, (b)T, (c)T, (d)F, (e)T
19. (a)T, (b)T, (c)F, (d)T, (e)F
20. (a)F, (b)F, (c)F, (d)T, (e)T
21. (a)T, (b)T, (c)T, (d)F, (e)T
22. (a)F, (b)T, (c)T, (d)T, (e)T
23. (a)F, (b)T, (c)F, (d)T, (e)T
24. (a)T, (b)T, (c)F, (d)F, (e)T
25. (a)T, (b)F, (c)T, (d)F, (e)F

26. (a)F, (b)T, (c)F, (d)F, (e)T
27. (a)T, (b)T, (c)T, (d)T, (e)T
28. (a)T, (b)F, (c)T, (d)T, (e)T
29. (a)T, (b)T, (c)F, (d)F, (e)F
30. (a)F, (b)F, (c)F, (d)T, (e)T
31. (a)T, (b)T, (c)T, (d)F, (e)F
32. (a)T, (b)F, (c)F, (d)F, (e)F
33. (a)T, (b)T, (c)T, (d)T, (e)T
34. (a)F, (b)F, (c)T, (d)F, (e)T
35. (a)T, (b)T, (c)T, (d)F, (e)T
36. (a)F, (b)F, (c)T, (d)F, (e)F
37. (a)T, (b)T, (c)F, (d)T, (e)T
38. (a)F, (b)F, (c)T, (d)T, (e)T
39. (a)T, (b)F, (c)T, (d)F, (e)T
40. (a)F, (b)F, (c)F, (d)F, (e)F
41. (a)T, (b)F, (c)T, (d)F, (e)T
42. (a)F, (b)F, (c)T, (d)F, (e)T
43. (a)T, (b)F, (c)T, (d)T, (e)F
44. (a)T, (b)T, (c)T, (d)T, (e)F
45. (a)T, (b)F, (c)T, (d)F, (e)T
46. (a)T, (b)T, (c)F, (d)F, (e)F
47. (a)T, (b)T, (c)T, (d)F, (e)T
48. (a)F, (b)F, (c)T, (d)F, (e)T
49. (a)F, (b)T, (c)T, (d)T, (e)F
50. (a)T, (b)F, (c)F, (d)T, (e)F

SAQ Answers

1. Schneider's first-rank symptoms are as follows:
   - Auditory hallucinations—thought-echo, hearing thoughts spoken aloud, discussing or giving a running commentary on the patient, or originating from another part of the patient's body.
   - Delusions of thought-control—thought-insertion/withdrawal/broadcast.
   - Delusions of control—somatic passivity, passivity of impulse/affect/volition.
   - Delusional perception.

2. Refer to Fig. 5.4.

3. The features of alcohol-dependence syndrome are:
   - Compulsion to drink alcohol.
   - Stereotyped pattern of drinking.
   - Physiological withdrawal symptoms.
   - Tolerance.
   - Neglect of other interests.
   - Reinstatement after abstinence.
     (three or more indicate dependence)

4. Personality is a person's enduring pattern of relating to the environment and thinking about themselves, across a wide range of personal and social contexts.
   To diagnose a personality disorder, the patient must be shown to have marked deviations in behaviour and attitudes from expected cultural norms which:
   - Are enduring and consistent across a range of personal experiences.
   - Have their origin in childhood and adolescence.
   - Cause distress to the patient or to others, leading to problems in social and personal functioning.

5. The main primary neurodegenerative causes of dementia are: Alzheimer's disease, vascular dementia, diffuse Lewy body dementia, Pick's disease, Huntington's disease, Creutzfeldt–Jakob disease, and HIV dementia. In addition, there are many general medical (sometimes treatable) causes (see Fig. 6.3).

6. Puerperal psychoses occur in 0.2% of women in the year after childbirth. Typically they are of rapid onset with considerable variation and intensity of symptoms. Disorientation and other signs of clouding of consciousness occur, which necessitates careful exclusion of a delirium. Schizophrenia has almost a 1% lifetime incidence; episodes normally last for several months after a gradual onset (often there are non-specific prodromal symptoms), and are chronic in a large proportion. Unlike puerperal psychosis, negative symptoms are common. Clouding of consciousness and disorientation are not typical; if they do occur an organic psychosis or delirium should be suspected. Both puerperal psychosis and schizophrenia may present with first rank symptoms, and both have a high risk of suicide.

7. Psychiatric disorders of childhood and adolescence are classified as follows:
   A. Developmental disorders:
   - Mental retardation (global learning disability).
   - Specific developmental disorders, e.g. reading delay.
   - Pervasive development disorders, e.g. autism.

   B. Acquired disorders:
   - Disorders usually specific to childhood, e.g. conduct disorder, hyperkinetic disorder.
   - Disorders usually presenting in adults, e.g. dementia, schizophrenia.

8. Categories of mental disorder included in the Mental Health Act 1983 are:
   - Mental illness.
   - Psychopathic disorder.
   - Mental impairment.
   - Severe mental impairment.

   Section 2 has a 28-day duration and the patient may appeal in the first 14 days. It is usually used for assessment if the diagnosis and likely response to treatment are unknown.
   Section 3 has a 6-month duration and the patient may appeal at any time. It is used for treatment of a mental disorder (ideally a treatment plan should be known beforehand). Patients with psychopathic disorder and mental impairment can only be detained if the proposed treatment is thought to alleviate the condition or prevent deterioration.

9. Principles of delirium management are:
   - Investigate and treat any underlying medical condition.
   - Try to nurse in a well-lit, quiet environment.
   - Maximize sensory function.
   - Encourage orientation of the patient.
   - If the disturbance requires sedative medication, low doses of haloperidol, trifluoperazine, or benzodiazepines are preferable.

10. Formal thought-disorder is an abnormality of the mechanism of thinking, which is almost always deduced (indirectly) by careful observation of a patient's speech.
    Several types are recognized:
    - Speed-of-thought abnormalities—flight of ideas, retardation.
    - Interruptions in the flow of thought—thought-blocking, derailment ('knights move thinking'), leading to word salad, verbigeration, crowding of thought, perseveration.

    Others:
    - Concrete thinking.
    - Neologisms.

11. The three main classes of antidepressants are:
    - Tricyclic agents (TCAs).
    - Selective serotonin reuptake inhibitors (SSRIs).
    - Monoamine oxidase inhibitors (MAOIs).

    TCAs often cause anticholinergic side effects such as dry mouth, blurred vision, constipation, and, sometimes, difficulty in micturition or urinary retention. Other common side effects include sedation, postural hypotension, dizziness, sexual dysfunction, and weight gain.
    SSRIs may cause nausea, headache, gastrointestinal disturbance, and abdominal pain. Some SSRIs are associated with insomnia, and increased anxiety and agitation in the early stages of treatment. Sexual dysfunction may also occur.
    The most common side effects attributable to MAOIs are postural hypotension and dizziness. Sleep problems or fatigue, dry mouth, constipation, blurred vision, headache, and agitation are among the other potential side effects of these agents.

12. 'Free-floating anxiety' is the experience of anxiety symptoms that are not tied exclusively to one specific situation or definite known external threat. Symptoms may arrive in any situation and may be persistent for hours or days.
    Generalized anxiety disorder, in which free-floating anxiety is a key feature, may be treated by medications or non-drug treatments.
    Drug treatments include:
    - Benzodiazepines (short term use).
    - Antipsychotics (short-term use for severe anxiety).
    - Buspirone.
    - Beta blockers (mainly for relief of autonomic anxiety symptoms).

    Non-drug treatments include:
    - Supportive therapy.
    - Cognitive–behavioural therapy.
    - Psychodynamic therapy.

13. As in all personality disorders, the dysfunctional personality should have its roots in adolescence or childhood, be fairly constant over a number of years, and produce a pattern recognizable to others. In borderline personality disorder, the behaviour pattern may involve:
    - Uncertain self-image and chronic feeling of emptiness.
    - Impulsive behaviour with ignorance of its consequences.
    - Unstable relationships.
    - Unstable mood.
    - Fear of abandonment.
    - Anger and violence towards others, or threats of, or actual, self-harm.

    Treatment of borderline personality disorder, whether by drug therapy or psychotherapy is difficult. In the short term, drugs may be used to control certain symptoms (e.g. benzodiazepines for anxiety, antipsychotics for anger), but underlying personality traits are usually resistant to change. In some cases, long term cognitive–behavioural therapy may eventually effect change.

14. Anhedonia is the inability to derive pleasure from activities that were previously enjoyed.
    Further biological (somatic) symptoms of depression include:
    - Appetite loss.
    - Poor self-esteem/worthlessness/uselessness.
    - Early morning wakening.
    - Loss of libido.
    - Diurnal variation in mood.
    - Reduced emotional reactivity.
    - Psychomotor retardation or agitation.

    Cognitive symptoms of depression include:
    - Poor concentration.
    - Poor self-esteem.
    - Guilt.
    - Hopelessness.
    - Suicidal ideation (although strictly speaking this is a cognitive symptom of depression, it is usually considered separately owing to its considerable importance).

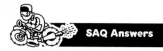

15. Obsessions are recurrent and persistent ideas, impulses, and images which are experienced as intrusive and inappropriate and cause marked anxiety and distress. They are recognized as being the individual's own thoughts and may provoke attempts at resistance but may be impossible to remove.

Compulsions are recurrent and persistent behaviours or mental acts undertaken to prevent or reduce anxiety or distress, usually through the belief that they will prevent a dreaded event from occurring. They do not produce pleasure or gratification, nor do the tasks they involve bring useful results, but if they are resisted, anxiety levels may increase.

Obsessional thoughts and compulsive acts that commonly occur together are:
- Thoughts of contamination associated with recurrent hand washing or avoidance of dust or germs.
- Obsessional doubt associated with repeated checking.
- A need for symmetry associated with compulsive slowness in maintaining symmetry.

16. Whilst the diagnosis of anorexia nervosa demands that patients are grossly underweight, there is no minimum weight for bulimic patients—their weight may in fact be normal. This means that changes associated with severe weight loss such as amenorrhoea are usually seen only in anorexia nervosa. Anorexia nervosa is associated with excessive control over eating but bulimia nervosa signals a loss of control, and binge eating is essential to the diagnosis only in the latter.

Weight loss may occur in the following psychiatric disorders:
- Affective disorders, including depression and bipolar affective disorder.
- Obsessive–compulsive disorder.
- Psychotic disorders (but antipsychotic drugs may cause weight gain).
- Alcohol and substance abuse.

Medical conditions that may be associated with weight loss include:
- Malignancies.
- Addison's disease.
- Inflammatory bowel disease (Crohn's, ulcerative colitis).
- Malabsorption.
- Diabetes mellitus.
- Hyperthyroidism.

17. a) Suicide (or 'completed suicide') has a fatal outcome, whereas in parasuicide the individual survives. Note that the term 'parasuicide' is applied to any suicide attempt that does not result in death irrespective of whether the individual intended to die or merely to draw attention to his or her problems.

b) In parasuicide the individual follows a course of action that could conceivably result in his or her death. Deliberate self-harm is a broader term, encompassing a spectrum of actions—from inflicting a minor injury (e.g. superficial cuts to the forearm), to performing a parasuicide with serious suicidal intent (e.g. jumping from a third-floor balcony but sustaining only a wrist fracture).

Psychiatric illnesses associated with suicide include:
- Depression.
- Alcohol and substance abuse.
- Schizophrenia.
- Personality disorders (e.g. borderline, antisocial).
- Panic disorder.
- Anorexia nervosa.

18. Psychiatric syndromes associated with the puerperium are:
- 'Baby blues'.
- Postnatal depression.
- Puerperal psychosis.

'Baby blues' occurs after one-third to one-half of pregnancies and requires no treatment other than reassurance and normal postpartum support.

Postnatal depression occurs after one in eight pregnancies. It should be treated with antidepressants and, if necessary, counselling. Note that antidepressants should be used with caution if the mother is breastfeeding.

Puerperal psychosis occurs after only 1 in 500 pregnancies. It is a psychiatric emergency which may require separation of mother and baby. Early prescription of antidepressants and antipsychotics is usually advisable. Lithium may be introduced—provided breastfeeding is avoided—if the psychosis is thought to be associated with a manic episode.

19. The patient has depression that has proved resistant to treatment after trials with two categories of antidepressant drugs at therapeutic doses for adequate time. The advantage of lithium augmentation is that the likelihood of providing a remission of symptoms is greater than that if a third antidepressant was tried.

The disadvantages are:

- Inconvenience—establishment of lithium therapy will require extra visits to the clinic and regular blood tests (including urea, electrolytes, and other baseline measures, as well as subsequent lithium levels). It also makes for a more complex drug regimen for the patient, who will have to take two drugs (lithium + tricyclic), rather than one.
- Side effects—lithium may cause numerous adverse effects such as tremor, gastrointestinal disturbance, polyuria, polydipsia, weight gain, thyroid problems, and cardiac arrhythmias.
- Toxicity—if lithium plasma levels exceed the upper end of the therapeutic range, toxic effects may ensue. These may include tremor, diarrhoea, vomiting, dysarthria, ataxia proceeding to muscle fasciculations, loss of consciousness, and seizures.

20. Panic-attack symptoms include:
- Palpitations.
- Nausea/abdominal distress.
- Sweating.
- Dizziness/feeling faint.
- Trembling.
- Derealization.
- Dry mouth.
- Depersonalization.
- Shortness of breath.
- Fear of losing control or dying.
- Choking sensation.
- Hot flushes/cold chills.
- Chest pain.
- Numbness/tingling.

To diagnose panic disorder there should be recurrent panic attacks (discrete episodes with four or more of these symptoms) which start abruptly and reach a peak quickly. Some or all of the attacks must be unexpected rather than occurring only in specific circumstances, and attacks must not be caused directly by a medical condition or substance. Note that DSM-IV requires that at least one attack is followed by persistent anticipatory anxiety, worry about its implications, or significant behavioural change.

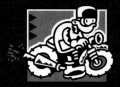

Index

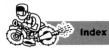

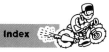

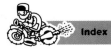

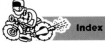

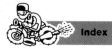

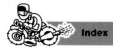

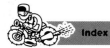

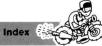